HA

OBSTETRICAL

EMERGENCIES

HANDBOOK OF

OBSTETRICAL

EMERGENCIES

Constance Sinclair
MSN, CNM, CEN
Redwood Midwifery Services
Santa Rosa, California
Critical Care Staff Nurse
Palm Drive Hospital
Sebastopol, California

W.B. SAUNDERS COMPANY
A Division of Harcourt Brace & Company
Philadelphia London Toronto
Montreal Sydney Tokyo

W.B. SAUNDERS COMPANY
A Division of Harcourt Brace & Company

The Curtis Center
Independence Square West
Philadelphia, Pennsylvania 19106

Library of Congress Cataloging-in-Publication Data

Sinclair, Constance.
Handbook of obstetrical emergencies / Constance Sinclair.—
    1st ed.

p.   cm.

ISBN 0–7216–6431–8

1. Obstetrical emergencies—Handbooks, manuals, etc.
    I. Title. [DNLM: 1. Pregnancy Complications—
    handbooks.   2. Labor Complications–handbooks.
    3. Obstetrics– handbooks.   4. Emergencies–
    handbooks.   WQ 39 S616h 1996]

RG571.S56 1996   618.2'025–dc20

DNLM/DLC   95-52229

HANDBOOK OF
OBSTETRICAL EMERGENCIES   ISBN 0–7216–6431–8

Printed in the United States of America.

Last digit is the print number: 9   8   7   6   5   4   3   2   1

*To the staff of the Emergency Department
of The Graduate Hospital of Philadelphia, Pennsylvania.
In the beginning, you were my teachers.
You became my friends,
and then my family and my home.*

*And to Steve, Hannah, and Olivia.
Because of you, I know heaven.*

REVIEWERS

KATHY DeBROCK CLARKE, RNC
Office of Michael S. Phillips, MD
Richardson, Texas

MARY FRANCES DAMPIER, MD, PhD
Emergency Department Physician,
Paoli Memorial Hospital
Paoli, Pennsylvania

LINDA VALERIE HACKLEY, RN, MS, CEN
Swedish Medical Center
Englewood, Colorado

LINELL JONES, RN, BSN, CEN, CCRN
Department of Emergency Services
Valley Medical Center
Renton, Washington

JOHN LAWRIE, MD, FACEP
Medical Director, Emergency Department
The Graduate Hospital
Philadelphia, Pennsylvania

JAMES B. RICHMANN, RN, BS, CEN, ENPC-I
Nursing Department Head of Emergency Services
Our Lady of Lourdes Medical Center
Camden, New Jersey

SUZANNE R. SCHOENECKER, RN, CEN
Nurse Manager, Emergency Department
The Graduate Hospital
Philadelphia, Pennsylvania

PREFACE

Handbook of Obstetrical Emergencies provides the user with easily accessible basic guidelines for the nursing assessment and care of the pregnant patient experiencing an obstetrical emergency. Emergency nurses, new obstetrical nurses, student nurses, paramedics, medical students, and nurse-midwifery students will find this information useful. The handbook may be used for orientation, for the development of protocols, and for the delivery drills that most emergency departments conduct periodically. The medical interventions suggested in this handbook should be covered by institutional protocols and/or by the order of a nurse-midwife, a nurse-practitioner, or a physician.

Institutions may or may not have an in-house labor and delivery unit to which pregnant patients may be transferred or from which obstetrical nurses, nurse-midwives, or obstetricians might be called to the emergency department. Hospitals with an obstetrical department should have policies regarding when the patient receives care in the emergency department and when she receives care in labor and delivery. In hospitals without an obstetrical department, when transfer to an obstetrical department involves transfer to another facility, policies must be in place to identify the timing of such a transfer. In implementing the policy in each case, the risk of maternal or fetal deterioration in transport must be weighed against the need for immediate obstetrical attendance. This book addresses both of these hospital situations.

Electronic fetal monitoring (EFM) is a vital assessment tool in the obstetrical unit. Interpretation of EFM, however, is a complex skill that is in the domain of obstetrical, and not emergency, nurses. Use of EFM without proper training presents a litigious risk to emergency staff. In a hospital with an obstetrical department, a fetal monitor may be brought to the emergency department for evaluation and observation of a patient, but an obstetrical nurse or an obstetrician must be continuously present and responsible for its interpretation. EFM interpretation, therefore, is not included in this handbook. The interpretation of fetal heart tone variations that can be auscultated by Doppler or fetoscope is discussed.

Finally, birth is a normal event that is ideally conducted with as little intervention as possible, where the miracle of birth and the family are the focus. However, a birth that occurs in the emergency department is, in most cases, one for which the mother has had no prenatal care or one in which the labor has been precipitous. Each of these situations presents risks for the mother and for the fetus. The paramount concern is the safety of the mother and baby. Safeguards such as oxygen administration and intravenous access are therefore included in the guidelines for normal birth in this handbook.

This handbook is meant to be portable for convenient use on the job. The information included is brief and action-oriented. For more comprehensive information regarding the subject matter, the following resources are suggested:

Chameides, L., & Hazinski, M. F. (Eds.). (1994). *Textbook of pediatric advanced life support.* Dallas: American Heart Association and American Academy of Pediatrics.

Cunningham, F. G., et al. (1993). *Williams obstetrics* (19th ed.). Norwalk, CT: Appleton & Lange.

La Leche League. (1991). *The womanly art of breastfeeding* (5th rev. ed.). New York: Penguin Books.

Parer, J. T. (1983). *Handbook of fetal heart rate monitoring.* Philadelphia: W. B. Saunders Co.

Star, W. L., Lommel, L. L., & Shannon, M. T. (1995). *Women's primary health care: Protocols for practice.* Waldorf, MD: American Nurses Publishing.

ACKNOWLEDGMENTS

I am indebted to Sue Schoenecker, who supported my idea to write this book. I am particularly grateful for the input from Jim Richmann, my emergency nurse role model; and from Mary Frances Dampier, physician extraordinaire. Special thanks to Ilze Rader at the W.B. Saunders Company, who first expressed interest in the manuscript; and to Barbara Nelson Cullen, my editor at W.B. Saunders, who made this publishing experience a pleasurable one.

NOTICE

Emergency nursing is an ever-changing field. Standard safety precautions must be followed, but as new research and clinical experience broaden our knowledge, changes in treatment and drug therapy become necessary or appropriate. The editors of this work have carefully checked the generic and trade drug names and verified drug dosages to ensure that the dosage information in this work is accurate and in accord with the standards accepted at the time of publication. Readers are advised, however, to check the product information currently provided by the manufacturer of each drug to be administered to be certain that changes have not been made in the recommended dose or in the contraindications for administration. This is of particular importance in regard to new or infrequently used drugs. It is the responsibility of the treating physician, relying on experience and knowledge of the patient, to determine dosages and the best treatment for the patient. The editors cannot be responsible for misuse or misapplication of the material in this work.

THE PUBLISHER

CONTENTS

Terbutaline (Brethine) 96
Vitamin K (AquaMEPHYTON) 97

APPENDICES

Apendix A

Appendix B

Appendix C

Appendix D

Appendix E

Appendix F

Appendix G

Appendix H

Normal Pregnancy: Description and Assessment

ASSESSING GESTATIONAL AGE

Assessing Gestational Age by Naegele's Rule

Pregnancy is considered to last approximately 280 days (40 weeks) from the first day of the last normal menstrual period (LNMP or LMP). A normal menstrual period is one typical of the woman's usual cycles in timing, duration, amount of flow, and amount of cramping. This definition of pregnancy includes the menses, the time of ovum preparation until ovulation, and actual conception at approximately 14 days. Traditionally the due date (*expected date of confinement* [EDC] or the *expected date of delivery* [EDD]) is calculated by *Naegele's rule* as follows: Identify the first day of the LNMP, add 7 days, and subtract 3 months. Alternatively, the pregnancy wheel, set with the appropriate arrow on the LNMP, gives the EDC within 1 to 3 days. Continuing to use the wheel, look at the present date to find the number of weeks' gestation. This method is less accurate if the patient is uncertain of the LNMP, if the normalcy of that menses is questionable, if the woman's cycle is usually irregular, if the woman recently used a hormonal method of birth control, if the woman is or was recently lactating, or if the woman is perimenopausal.

Assessing Gestational Age by Ultrasound

Ultrasound determination of gestational age between 7 and 14 weeks' gestation (by crown-rump measurement) is accurate ±4.7 days, between 12 and 22 weeks' gestation (by measurement of femur length) is accurate ±6.7 days, and between 17 and 26 weeks (by measurement of the biparietal diameter

[BPD] of the fetal skull) is accurate ±10 days. After 26 weeks, gestational age determination is made by BPD and is accurate ±2 to 3 weeks (Cunningham et al., 1993).

Assessing Gestational Age by Fundal Height

Figure 1–1 illustrates fundal height (the top of the uterus) throughout pregnancy. This figure assumes that the bladder is empty and that the woman is average in height and trunk proportions. The figure assumes a single fetus of average size and, in the last few weeks, assumes a vertex (head-down) position. During the last month, the measurement may stay at about the 36-week height as the fetus continues to grow while settling down into the pelvis in preparation for delivery (known as engagement or "dropping").

Assessing Gestational Age by Laboratory Tests

A serum qualitative human chorionic gonadotropin (hCG) is positive 8 to 9 days after ovulation. A urine hCG is positive a few days after the missed menses (Cunningham et al., 1989). The serum quantitative hCG is a measurement of the amount of hCG, which, in a healthy pregnancy, increases until the second to third month, when it plateaus. See Table 1–1 for levels of hCG (and other normal laboratory findings) that can be expected at different points during pregnancy.

"Soft" Indicators of Gestational Age

Fetal heart tones are audible by fetoscope (as opposed to Doppler) at approximately 17 to 19 weeks' gestation (Cunningham et al., 1993).

The primigravida feels fetal movement ("quickening") at approximately 20 weeks' gestation, whereas the multigravida recognizes movement at approximately 18 weeks' gestation. This marker is, however, highly variable.

TRIMESTERS OF PREGNANCY

Pregnancy is often described by trimesters, three periods of 3 months each:

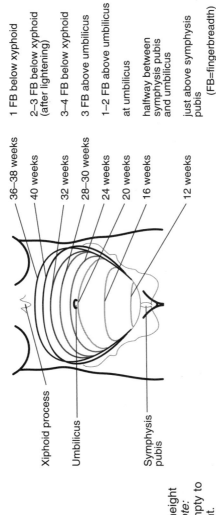

Figure 1–1. Fundal height during pregnancy. *Note:* Bladder should be empty to measure fundal height.

36–38 weeks — 1 FB below xyphoid

40 weeks — 2–3 FB below xyphoid (after lightening)

32 weeks — 3–4 FB below xyphoid

28–30 weeks — 3 FB above umbilicus

24 weeks — 1–2 FB above umbilicus

20 weeks — at umbilicus

16 weeks — halfway between symphysis pubis and umbilicus

12 weeks — just above symphysis pubis

(FB=fingerbreadth)

Xiphoid process

Umbilicus

Symphysis pubis

Table 1-1. Normal Laboratory Findings in Pregnancy*

	Nonpregnant Woman	Pregnant Woman
RBC†		
Hematocrit	37–48%	32–42%
Hemoglobin	12–16 g/dL	10–14 g/dL
WBC	4500–10,000 mm	5000–14,000 mm
Platelets	150,000–350,000	Normal or slightly decreased
Fibrinogen	300 mg/100 mL	600 mg/100 mL
PT†	12–15 sec ±2 sec control	Slightly shortened
Ptt†	25–37 sec	Slightly shortened
BUN	10–18 mg/dL	4–12 mg/dL
Creatinine	0.6–1.2 mg	0.4–0.9 mg
Creatinine clearance	3.5–5.0 mL/min	2.0–3.5 mL/min
Alkaline phosphatase	13–35 IU/mL	25–80 IU/mL
Albumin	3.5–5.0 g/dL	3.0–4.5 g/dL
ESR†	0–20 mm/hr	Strikingly elevated
Fasting glucose		
Serum	70–110 mg/dL	Unchanged
Whole blood	60–100 mg/dL	Unchanged
Na	135–145 mEq/L	132–140 mEq/L
K	3.5–5.0 mEq/L	3.5–4.5 mEq/L

Cl	100–106 mEq/L	90–105 mEq/L
HCO₃	24–30 mEq/L	17–22 mEq/L
Indirect Coombs	Negative	Negative
Urinalysis[†]	Negative	1/6 all pregnant women have glycosuria
Qualitative hCG	Negative	Positive a few days after missed menses
Quantitative hCG[‡]	0–3 mIU/mL	preg. 1 wk	5–50 IU/mL
		2 wk	40–200 IU/mL
		3 wk	100–500 IU/mL
		4 wk	700–2000 IU/mL
		2–3 mo	12,000–200,000 IU/mL
		2nd trimester	24,000–55,000 IU/mL
		3rd trimester	6000–48,000 IU/mL
Arterial blood gases			
pH	7.38–7.44	7.41–7.46
PO_2	95–100 mm Hg	100–108 mm Hg
PCO_2	35–45 mm Hg	27–32 mm Hg
HCO₃	24–30 mM/L	19–25 mM/L
Base excess	0.7 mEq/L	3–4 mEq/L
Electrocardiogram		Flattened or inverted T waves may be seen in leads III, V_1, and V_2, and Q waves may be seen in leads III and AVF because of left deviation of the electrical axis as the heart is displaced up and forward

* Data from Esposito, 1994.
† Data from Cunningham et al., 1993.
‡ *Note:* If quantitative hCG is 1053 IU/mL or more, fetal pole should be visible by ultrasound.

First trimester—first 12 weeks of pregnancy.
Second trimester—13–27 weeks' gestation.
Third trimester—28 weeks until delivery.

See Table 1–2 for changes during a normal pregnancy in each trimester.

GRAVIDITY AND PARITY

Gravidity is the number of times a woman has been pregnant. Most commonly, *parity* refers to the number of pregnancies that resulted in the birth of a fetus that reached viability (28 weeks). For example, the woman who has been pregnant four times, has had one miscarriage at 10 weeks, has had two full-term deliveries, and is presently pregnant would be described as a gravida 4, para 2 (Gr 4 P 2).

A more thorough designation of parity, although used less commonly, is expressed in four numbers. The first is the number of infants born at full-term; the second is the number of infants born prematurely; the third is the number of abortions (spontaneous or induced); and the fourth is the number of children who are presently alive. In the example given, if the two infants born at full-term were still alive, the woman would be designated as a Gr 4 P 2012.

AUSCULTATION OF FETAL HEART TONES

Indication

Auscultation of fetal heart tones (FHTs) is done for reassurance of fetal well-being from 9 to 12 weeks' gestation by Doppler and by Doppler or fetoscope from 20 weeks until delivery.

Technique

The best instrument for auscultating FHTs in the emergency department (E.D.) is a Doppler with a digital display of the beat-to-beat rate. Determine the fetal position and listen over the fetal shoulder to hear best. If using a fetoscope or a Doppler without the digital display, listen to the heart for 5-second intervals and multiply by 12, determining the rate for each 5-second interval heard. If the woman is having uterine con-

Table 1–2. Changes During Normal Pregnancy

First Trimester

- Conception occurs on approximately the 14th day of the menstrual cycle
- Blastocyst (the developing fertilized ovum) implants in the uterus 8 to 9 days after conception, sometimes accompanied by a small amount of painless bleeding, which may be misinterpreted as a menstrual period
- Serum hCG becomes positive after implantation, on days 22 to 23 of the menstrual cycle
- Menstrual period is missed
- A few days after the missed menses, the urine hCG becomes positive
- Early first-trimester blood pressure reflects prepregnancy values (Sibai and Mabie, 1991)
- Breast tingling and tenderness begin
- Nausea and vomiting may occur
- Fatigue may occur
- Urinary frequency occurs
- Uterus enlarges, becomes globular in shape, softens, and flexes easily over the cervix
- Cervix softens (Goodell's sign) and becomes bluish purple (Chadwick's sign)
- FHTs may be heard by Doppler between 9 and 12 weeks
- Uterus can be palpated just above the symphysis pubis at approximately 12 weeks (see Fig. 1–1)
- In late first trimester, blood pressure begins to drop as a result of hormonally mediated decreased resistance in the peripheral vascular bed (Sibai and Mabie, 1991)
- By 12 weeks, the embryonic period of fetal development ends, organogenesis being complete, with growth and maturation of fetal organs continuing in the second and third trimesters

Second Trimester

- By weeks 12 to 16, nausea, vomiting, fatigue, and urinary frequency of the first trimester improve
- The mother recognizes fetal movement ("quickening") at approximately 18 to 20 weeks (the multigravida earlier)
- Veins of the breast enlarge and are more visible through the skin. Breasts enlarge, and areola and nipples darken. Colostrum may be expressed from the nipples
- Midline of the abdominal skin becomes pigmented and is called the linea nigra
- Striae ("stretch marks") may be noted on breasts, abdomen, and areas of weight gain
- Systolic blood pressure may be 2 to 8 mm Hg lower and diastolic blood pressure 5 to 15 mm Hg lower than prepregnancy levels (Esposito, 1994). This drop may cause symptoms of dizziness and faintness, particularly after rising quickly
- Stomach displacement and altered esophageal and gastric tone predispose the woman to heartburn

Table continued on following page

Table 1–2. Changes During Normal Pregnancy *Continued*

Second Trimester

- Intestines are displaced, and tone and motility are decreased, often causing constipation
- Gallbladder may become distended and hypotonic, predisposing some women to gallstone formation
- Hormones act on the respiratory center in the brain to increase the respiratory drive. Respiratory rate changes little, but tidal volume increases as pregnancy advances. This causes a slight drop in $Paco_2$, causing a mild respiratory alkalosis (Cunningham et al., 1993)
- Thyroid gland enlarges
- Gums may hypertrophy and bleed easily
- Nosebleeds may occur more frequently
- FHTs are audible by fetoscope (as opposed to Doppler) at about 17 to 19 weeks
- Fetal outline is palpable through the abdominal wall at approximately 20 weeks
- At 28 weeks, fetus is considered viable
- See Figure 1–1 for growth of the uterine fundus during the second trimester

Third Trimester

- Blood volume, which increased rapidly during the second trimester, peaks at 30 weeks to an amount approximately 45% greater than the prepregnancy level and plateaus thereafter. Plasma increases by about 48% and erythrocytes by about 33%, causing a slight hemodilution and a small drop in hematocrit (Cunningham et al., 1993)
- Blood pressure slowly rises again to approximately the prepregnant level (Sibai and Mabie, 1991)
- Uterine enlargement causes the diaphragm to rise and the shape of the rib cage to widen at the base. Decreased space for lung expansion may cause a sense of shortness of breath
- Heart is displaced by the rising diaphragm up and to the left. Cardiac output, stroke volume, and force of contraction are increased (Cunningham et al., 1993). Pulse rate rises by 10 to 15 bpm (Cunningham et al., 1993). A systolic murmur can be heard in 90% of pregnant women (Cunningham et al., 1993)
- Edema of the lower extremities may occur, worsening with dependency, such as prolonged standing
- Varicosities, if present, enlarge due to vascular relaxation as well as engorgement caused by the weight of the full uterus compressing the vessels of the pelvic area
- Hemorrhoids, varicosities of the rectum, may occur as discussed above, and secondary to constipation
- Progressive lordosis occurs to compensate for the shifting center of balance caused by the anteriorly bulging uterus, predisposing the woman to backaches. Associated slumping of the shoulders and

Table 1–2. Changes During Normal Pregnancy *Continued*

Third Trimester

anterior flexion of the neck may cause aching and numbness of the arms and hands
- Approximately 2 weeks before going into labor, the primigravida experiences engagement (also called "lightening" or "dropping"), when the vertex moves down into the pelvis. Symptoms include a lower appearing fundus, urinary frequency, increased vaginal secretions, and increased lung capacity. In the multigravida, the fetus may move down at any time in late pregnancy or often not until labor
- Fundal height increases to a fingerbreadth below the xiphoid process at 36 weeks and may drop by 2 to 3 fingerbreadths when engagement occurs (see Fig. 1–1)
- Cervical effacement and dilation begin
- The mucus plug is expelled at variable times before or during labor
- Between 37 and 42 weeks, the pregnancy is considered full-term. After 42 weeks, the pregnancy is considered postdates

tractions, listen before the contraction to determine the baseline rate, listen during the contraction, and listen for 1 minute after the contraction. In the third trimester, observe fetal movement (or elicit it) and listen to the fetal heart tones for 30 seconds afterward (Fig. 1–2). Fetal movement may be elicited by gently moving the fetus through the abdominal wall (the mother may be able to do this for you). Having the mother drink oral fluids or doing a vaginal examination may also elicit fetal movements if either measure is appropriate.

Descriptions of Auscultated Fetal Heart Tone Patterns

Baseline Rate. The average rate occurring between uterine contractions when there are no accelerations or decelerations. The normal FHT baseline is between 120 and 160 beats per minute (bpm).

Mild Bradycardia. Baseline rate 100 to 119 bpm; not necessarily evidence of fetal hypoxemia (Cunningham et al., 1993).

Marked Bradycardia. Baseline rate 99 bpm or less; cause for serious concern. It may occur with fetal acidosis, congenital heart lesions, or marked maternal hypothermia (Cunningham et al., 1993).

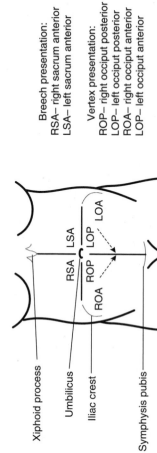

Breech presentation:
RSA– right sacrum anterior
LSA– left sacrum anterior

Vertex presentation:
ROP– right occiput posterior
LOP– left occiput posterior
ROA– right occiput anterior
LOP– left occiput anterior

Xiphoid process

Umbilicus

Iliac crest

Symphysis pubis

Figure 1–2. Locations for the auscultation of fetal heart tones in the third trimester.

▶ Important Note:*Verify that the rate heard is not the maternal heart rate (synchronous with the maternal radial pulse).*

Tachycardia. Persistent baseline greater than 180 bpm. It usually occurs in the presence of maternal fever; may occur with maternal drug ingestion, fetal infection, maternal thyrotoxicosis, or fetal anemia, and rarely is diagnosed as a fetal arrhythmia (Gabbe et al., 1991).

Decelerations. Decrease in heart rate below baseline. Decelerations are worrisome if they have the following characteristics:

- A drop to 80 bpm or lower regardless of duration.
- More than 30 seconds in duration regardless of depth of deceleration.
- Recurring persistently.
- Occurring regularly after the peak or conclusion of a contraction—even a subtle drop such as 5 bpm is significant (Gabbe et al., 1991).

Accelerations. Increase in the rate higher than the baseline. An acceleration of at least 15 bpm, lasting 15 seconds or more, occurring twice in a 10- to 15-minute period is generally considered a reassuring sign of fetal well-being (Cunningham et al., 1993).

For a description of auscultated fetal heart tones during delivery, please see page 52.

PALPATION OF UTERINE CONTRACTIONS

To assess uterine contractions, in addition to eliciting the patient's description, gently rest the palmar surface of the hand on the fundus of the uterus (Fig. 1–3). When the uterus contracts, your hand will be lifted and your fingers will be drawn closer together. As the contraction ebbs, the uterus will lower and your fingers will assume their original configuration. To judge the strength of the contractions, gently press the uterus with your fingertips in several places to gauge its "indentability." During a mild contraction, the uterus can be indented and feels like the tip of your nose. During a moder-

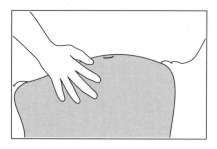

A Uterus at rest
(note hand resting on uterus
with fingers spread).

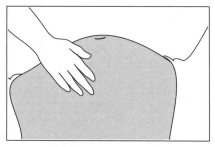

B Contracted uterus
(note hand still resting on uterus with
fingers now drawn together).

Figure 1–3. *A* and *B,* Palpation of uterine contractions.

ate contraction, the uterus feels like a chin. During strong contractions, the uterus is unyielding and feels as hard as your forehead.

TIMING OF UTERINE CONTRACTIONS

Count from the beginning of one contraction (as perceived by the mother or as palpated) to the beginning of the next contraction to determine interval. Note also the length of the contraction. Contractions may be irregular, so the timing should be observed for a series of contractions (Fig. 1–4).

Example:
These contractions are occurring
every three minutes, lasting
one minute each

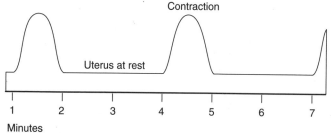

Figure 1–4. Timing of uterine contractions.

CERVICAL EXAMINATION

Indications

A cervical examination is performed to determine the dilation, effacement, location, and texture of the cervix and to determine fetal presenting part and station as well as the presence or absence of the umbilical cord at the cervix.

Technique

Using sterile gloves and lubricant (but not used before Nitrazine paper for determination of rupture of membranes; see p. 106), the examiner places the second and third fingers of the dominant hand into the vagina and assesses for effacement, dilation, and station.

Effacement. Thinning of the cervix. Before any changes occur in preparation for labor, the average cervix is between 2 and 3 cm long. The measurement is stated as a percentage, so a 2 cm long cervix is called uneffaced or 0% effaced. A 1 cm cervix is called 50% effaced. The 100% effaced cervix is paper thin. Effacement is estimated by placing your finger through the cervical canal and resting it on the presenting part, noting the depth of the cervix against your finger.

Dilation. The diameter of the opening of the cervical os. When the internal os measures differently than the external

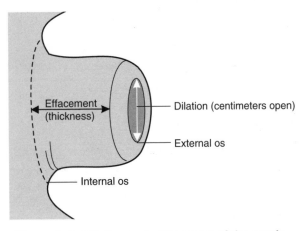

Figure 1–5. Dilation and effacement of the cervix.

os, both are noted. Dilation is measured in centimeters with 10 cm being complete dilation (Fig. 1–5). At complete dilation, the cervix is actually absent, and uterus and vagina have become a continuous muscular tube.

Station. The height of the presenting part in relation to the ischial spines of the pelvis. Station is expressed as a positive or negative number, which represents centimeters above (negative) or below (positive) the spines (Fig. 1–6).

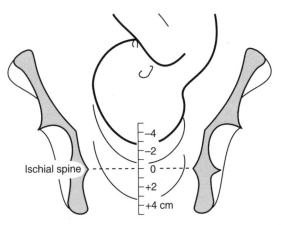

Figure 1–6. Cross section of the pelvis with a vertex at various stations.

Table 1–3 lists considerations for the assessment of the pregnant patient in an emergency.

Table 1–3. Assessment of the Pregnant Emergency Patient

I. Primary survey
  A. Presenting problem: onset, precipitating event
  B. Airway/cervical spine immobilization if appropriate
  C. Breathing
  D. Circulation: pulse, bleeding, and perfusion
II. Secondary survey
  A. Subjective data
    1. History of present illness or injury
      a. PQRST
        (1) Provocation of illness
        (2) Quality of symptoms
        (3) Region/radiation of problem
        (4) Severity of symptoms
        (5) Time of onset
      b. What makes it better or worse?
      c. Effect on daily activities?
      d. Patient's ideas about what is wrong
      e. What has patient tried?
      f. Has patient had this problem before?
      g. If trauma, mechanism of injury
    2. Family history, particularly hypertension, diabetes, and others relevant to the presenting problem
    3. Medical history including allergies
    4. Surgical history
    5. Obstetrical history, including the following information regarding each pregnancy:
      a. Month and year of delivery
      b. How many weeks' gestation
      c. Whether births were vaginal or cesarean
      d. Birth weight
      e. Complications
    6. Gynecological history
      a. Age at menarche, number of days in menstrual cycle, number of days of bleeding, quantity of bleeding, menstrual cramping
      b. Sexually transmitted diseases
      c. Abnormal Pap smears
      d. Whether currently sexually active
      e. If so, birth control method
    7. History of present pregnancy
      a. LNMP, EDC, and present weeks' gestation (see p. 1)
      b. Whether receiving prenatal care
      c. Illnesses during pregnancy
      d. Drugs and medications taken during pregnancy
      e. Complications of this pregnancy

Table continued on following page

Table 1–3. Assessment of the Pregnant Emergency Patient
Continued

  f. Is the fetus moving?
  g. Edema of ankles, face, hands; if present, onset
  h. Signs and symptoms of preeclampsia: headache, visual changes, sudden edema, epigastric pain, 5-lb weight gain in last week
  i. Signs and symptoms of urinary tract infection: dysuria, frequency, urgency, flank pain, fever, chills, nausea and vomiting, malaise
  j. Signs and symptoms of labor: contractions (onset, frequency, length, strength [can you walk and talk through them?]), loss of mucus plug, vaginal bleeding, rupture of membranes
 B. Objective data
  1. Head-to-toe physical assessment including:
   a. Breasts
    (1) Masses, nipple condition, discharge, lymph nodes, inflammation
   b. Abdomen
    (1) Fundal height (see p. 3)
    (2) Fetal position
    (3) Fetal movement
    (4) FHTs (see p. 6)
    (5) Uterine tenderness
    (6) Uterine contractions
    (7) Other abdominal mass
    (8) Abdominal pain or shoulder pain
    (9) Presence of bowel sounds
    (10) Hepatosplenomegaly
   c. Pelvis
    (1) Lymphatic nodes
    (2) Vaginal bleeding
    (3) External lesions
    (4) Vaginal secretions (? amniotic fluid; see p. 106)
    (5) Cervix: inflammation, lesions, friability, secretions, dilation, effacement, tenderness with motion, station, consistency
    (6) Uterus by bimanual palpation: tenderness, size, position
    (7) Adnexa: tenderness, mass
   d. Extremities: deep tendon reflexes, Homans' sign, varicosities, areas of swelling, redness, hardness, tenderness, and heat
III. Diagnostic procedures
 A. Laboratory
 B. Imaging: radiographs, ultrasound, computed tomography scan, magnetic resonance imaging
 C. Other procedures appropriate for presenting problem

Adapted from Blair, F. A., and Hall, M. M. (1994). The nursing process: Assessment and priority setting. In Klein, A. R., et al. (Eds.), Emergency Nursing Core Curriculum (pp. 3–23). Philadelphia: W.B. Saunders.

Complications of Pregnancy

ABORTION

Abortion is the termination of pregnancy by any means before the fetus is sufficiently developed to survive. Other commonly used definitions are the delivery of a fetus before 20 weeks' gestation or the delivery of a fetus less than 500 g (Cunningham et al., 1993). Approximately one third of all pregnancies end in abortions that occur before the pregnancy has been recognized. Of the pregnancies that are recognized, 12 to 26% spontaneously abort (Cunningham et al., 1993). Eighty percent of abortions occur in the first 12 weeks (Cunningham et al., 1993). In at least half of these, chromosomal anomalies are present. Other causes of abortion include systemic maternal disease, increasing parity, increasing maternal and paternal age, drug and environmental factors, uterine defects, and conception within 3 months of a live birth (Cunningham et al., 1993). There are six classifications of abortions: threatened, inevitable or incomplete, missed, complete, septic, and habitual or recurrent.

Miscarriage is a loss that, although minimized in our culture, must be resolved through the grieving process. Most women and their significant others struggle to understand why the loss occurred. Many women respond with guilt regarding recent activities that they fear caused the abortion, such as vacuuming or heavy lifting. They should be reassured that a healthy pregnancy withstands such activities without harm. Emotionally supportive care and appropriate referrals are required for the patient and her significant others. The patient should be advised to wait 3 months before attempting pregnancy again. The patient should be offered a birth control method before discharge.

The term *abortion* is used by the lay public to indicate an induced abortion, and the term should be used with sensitivity.

Threatened Abortion

Description. Vaginal bleeding during the first 20 weeks of an intrauterine pregnancy, which may or may not be accompanied by abdominal menstrual-like cramps or low back pain. The pregnancy may continue to term, or an abortion may occur. Between 20 and 40% of pregnant women experience vaginal spotting, and of these approximately half abort (Cunningham et al., 1993).

Clinical and Diagnostic Findings May Include

Signs and symptoms of pregnancy.
Vaginal bleeding (scant to profuse; brown, pink, or red).
Signs and symptoms of hypovolemic shock may be seen if the blood loss has been significant.
Uterine cramping (ominous).
Positive hCG, but the quantitative hCG may be less than expected for gestational age.
Uterus enlarged to size consistent with dates and may be tender.
Intact intrauterine pregnancy by ultrasound.
Closed cervical os.

Differential Diagnoses. Ectopic pregnancy, another category of abortion, cervicitis, vaginitis, cervical polyps, hydatidiform mole, implantation bleeding, cervical cancer, normal hyperemia of the pregnant cervix.

Nursing Actions

1. Maintain ABCs.
2. Observe vital signs and skin signs, and assess amount of vaginal bleeding.
3. If hemodynamically unstable, check pulse oximetry and administer supplemental oxygen if appropriate. Elevate patient's legs.
4. If hemodynamically unstable, initiate large-bore intravenous line with lactated Ringer's.
5. If hemodynamically unstable, or until the need for surgery is ruled out, keep patient NPO.
6. Draw blood for complete blood count (CBC), quantitative hCG, PT, Ptt, type, Rh, antibody

screen, and electrolytes, and hold blood for crossmatching (send for several units if unstable).

7. Anticipate gentle pelvic examination with cultures (including chlamydia and gonorrhea).
8. Anticipate ultrasound examination. If the patient is stable, she should begin drinking a large quantity of fluids to fill her bladder. If she is unstable, an indwelling urinary catheter should be placed to prepare the patient for ultrasound and to observe urine output.
9. Explain procedures and findings to the patient and her significant others. Offer emotional support for their potential loss.
10. The administration of $Rh_0(D)$ immune globulin after threatened abortion is controversial but may be ordered. Administer the microdose or include in instructions as below (see pp. 95–96).

Discharge Instructions. Instruct the patient to call her prenatal care provider immediately for follow-up. If she is not receiving prenatal care, make appropriate referrals.

If the patient is Rh-negative and $Rh_0(D)$ immune globulin has been ordered but not given, instruct the patient to contact her prenatal care provider to arrange to receive the medication within 72 hours.

The patient should seek immediate care for the following danger signs: fever, increased bleeding or cramping, or passage of tissue from vagina (saving the latter for examination by laboratory).

Pelvic rest (nothing in the vagina) is advised until the patient is released by her prenatal care provider.

Rest has not been proven to improve outcome but is generally implemented.

Inevitable or Incomplete Abortion

Description. Intrauterine pregnancy of less than 20 weeks' gestation with products of conception partially expelled. Pregnancy loss is certain. Heavy vaginal bleeding may cause hypovolemic shock. Sepsis (causative or secondary) may also occur.

Clinical and Diagnostic Findings May Include

Signs and symptoms of pregnancy.

Vaginal bleeding and possibly passage of tissue.

Signs and symptoms of hypovolemic shock may be
present if blood loss has been significant.

Uterine cramping.

Positive hCG.

Open cervical os.

Uterus enlarged and boggy; may be smaller than
expected for dates.

Remaining products of conception are intrauterine by
ultrasound (i.e., not ectopic).

Nitrazine-positive fluid may be coming from the os;
(i.e., amniotic fluid; see p. 106).

Differential Diagnoses. Ectopic pregnancy, other causes of
vaginal bleeding (see threatened abortion).

Nursing Actions

1. Maintain ABCs.
2. Assess vital signs and skin signs and amount of
   vaginal bleeding.
3. If hemodynamically unstable, check pulse
   oximetry and administer supplemental oxygen
   if appropriate. Elevate the patient's legs.
4. Keep the patient NPO.
5. Initiate large-bore intravenous line with
   lactated Ringer's.
6. Draw blood for CBC, quantitative hCG, PT, Ptt,
   type, Rh, and antibody screen (to determine
   need for $Rh_0(D)$ immune globulin). Obtain and
   send urine sample for urinalysis (prerequisite for
   surgery). If hemodynamically unstable, send
   blood for crossmatching and order several units.
7. Anticipate gentle pelvic examination with
   cultures (including chlamydia and gonorrhea).
8. Anticipate ultrasound examination.
9. Place indwelling urinary catheter to prepare the
   patient for ultrasound, to observe urine output
   if she is hemodynamically unstable, and to be
   ready for surgery.
10. Anticipate sending the patient to surgery and
    prepare necessary consent and checklist.

11. Explain procedures and findings to the patient and her significant others.
12. Offer emotional support for their loss.
13. If the client is Catholic, offer to baptize the products of conception or to call a priest to do so.
14. Send any products of conception to pathology.

Missed Abortion

Description. Intrauterine pregnancy of less than 20 weeks' gestation in which the fetus has been dead for 4 to 8 weeks or more but the uterus has failed to expel the products of conception.

Clinical and Diagnostic Findings

History of missed menses, possibly with vaginal spotting.
Signs and symptoms of pregnancy have regressed (such as nausea and breast changes).
Uterus smaller than expected by dates (fetal growth cessation followed by shrinkage).
hCG negative.
Ultrasound shows intrauterine products of conception without heart motion.

Differential Diagnoses. Ectopic pregnancy and other causes of vaginal bleeding (see Threatened Abortion).

Nursing Actions

1. Monitor vital signs, skin signs, and vaginal bleeding.
2. Keep patient NPO.
3. Anticipate gentle pelvic examination with cultures (including chlamydia and gonorrhea).
4. Anticipate ultrasound (fill bladder).
5. Place large-bore intravenous line with lactated Ringer's. Draw blood for CBC, hCG, PT, Ptt, type, Rh, and antibody screen (to determine the need for $Rh_0(D)$ immune globulin). Obtain and send urine sample for urinalysis.

6. Explain procedures and findings to patient and her significant others.
7. Offer emotional support for the patient and her significant others.
8. If patient is Catholic, offer to have the products of conception baptized and arrange with the surgical department.

Complete Abortion

Description. Intrauterine pregnancy of less than 20 weeks' gestation in which all of the products of conception are completely expelled by the uterus.

Clinical and Diagnostic Findings May Include

History of a confirmed pregnancy.
History of having passed tissue or blood (or both) vaginally.
Uterus small, nontender, tightly contracted.
Scant, nonodorous vaginal bleeding.
Afebrile.
Ultrasound shows no intrauterine products of conception as well as no ectopic pregnancy.

Differential Diagnoses. Ectopic pregnancy and other causes of vaginal bleeding (see threatened abortion).

Nursing Actions

1. Monitor vital signs, skin signs, and vaginal bleeding.
2. Keep patient NPO until the need for surgery is ruled out.
3. Draw blood for CBC, hCG, type, Rh, and antibody screen (to determine the need for $Rh_0(D)$ immune globulin). Obtain urine sample for urinalysis to send if surgery is required.
4. Anticipate pelvic examination with cultures (including gonorrhea and chlamydia).
5. Anticipate ultrasound examination (fill bladder).
6. If indicated, administer $Rh_0(D)$ immune globulin in the E.D. Otherwise, arrange for the patient to

obtain from prenatal care provider as instructed below (see pp. 95–96).
7. Explain procedures and findings to the patient and significant others. Give emotional support.
8. If client is Catholic and has brought the products of conception, offer to baptize them. Products of conception should then be sent to pathology.

Discharge Instructions. Some obstetricians perform a dilatation and curettage (D&C) on a patient with a complete abortion regardless of the clinical findings to prevent a small, undetected portion of the products of conception from causing sepsis and bleeding at home later.

If the patient is going home from the E.D., arrange for the patient to see her prenatal care provider for administration of Rh_0 (D) immune globulin, if indicated, within 72 hours (see pp. 95–96). If the patient has not been receiving prenatal care, give appropriate referrals.

The patient should seek care immediately for the following danger signs: increased vaginal bleeding or uterine cramping, fever, malaise, or malodorous vaginal discharge.

Septic Abortion

Description. Any form of abortion complicated by infection. The infection may be causative or secondary. Without appropriate antibiotic treatment, septic shock may develop as well as the hypovolemic shock that may occur secondary to blood loss.

Clinical and Diagnostic Findings May Include

Any type of abortion described previously.
Fever.
Malodorous vaginal discharge.
Uterus extremely tender to palpation.

Nursing Actions

1. As described previously for treatment of specific type of abortion.
2. Anticipate initiation of antibiotic therapy.
3. Observe for signs and symptoms of septic shock.

Habitual (or Recurrent) Abortion

Description. Three or more consecutive spontaneous abortions of any variety. Although there may be no common causative factor, the patient desiring pregnancy should be referred to a perinatologist or counseled to seek the care of a perinatologist when she is interested in pursuing pregnancy in the future. The rate of successful subsequent pregnancies is 70 to 90% (Cunningham et al., 1993).

COMPLICATIONS OF INDUCED ABORTION

Description

Induced abortion involves emptying the uterus of the products of conception by suction catheter or by D&C when performed legally before 12 weeks. For interruption of later pregnancy (such as for a fetal demise), intra-amniotic injection of 20% saline or 30% urea into the uterus or pharmacological induction of labor is done. Prostaglandins, oxytocin (Pitocin), or antiprogesterone RU486 may be used. Alternatively, hysterotomy or even hysterectomy may be performed by laparotomy. Illegal street abortions involve any assortment of instruments or drugs to interrupt the pregnancy.

Normal findings after an induced abortion include menses-like uterine cramps; menses-like nonodorous vaginal bleeding for 2 weeks, with continued spotting possible until the fourth week; lack of fever; uterus small and nontender on examination; a negative serum hCG 2 weeks postprocedure; pelvic rest (nothing in the vagina) for 1 week after the procedure; and, if Rh-negative, treatment with $Rh_0(D)$ immune globulin (see pp. 95–96) within 72 hours of the procedure.

Complications of any induced abortion include concurrent or singular, undiagnosed ectopic pregnancy; empty but infected uterus (endometritis); retained products of conception that are preventing contraction of the uterus, causing uterine bleeding and possible infection; failure of procedure (pregnancy intact); perforation of uterus and possibly other abdominal organs; and massive hemorrhage from laceration to cervix, uterus, or other pelvic structures. Such complications can cause hypovolemic or septic shock (or both).

Clinical and Diagnostic Findings

History of recent induced abortion.
Abdominal or low back pain (or both).
Vaginal bleeding, possibly malodorous.
Elevated WBC.
Hematocrit and hemoglobin may not reflect the
    amount of blood loss in an acute bleeding episode.
Fever, malaise.
Boggy, enlarged uterus.
Cervix open or closed.
Extreme pain on cervical motion.
Bleeding from cervical os or from lacerations.
Positive hCG.

Nursing Actions

1. Maintain ABCs.
2. Monitor vital signs, skin signs, and bleeding.
3. If hemodynamically unstable, check pulse
   oximetry and administer supplemental oxygen if
   appropriate. Elevate the patient's legs.
4. If hemodynamically unstable, initiate large-bore
   intravenous line with lactated Ringer's.
5. Draw blood for CBC and quantitative PT, Ptt,
   hCG, and hold blood for crossmatching. Obtain
   urine sample for urinalysis in case surgery is
   required. Type, Rh, and antibody screen should
   be ordered in the patient who might require
   $Rh_0(D)$ immune globulin.
6. Anticipate gentle pelvic examination with
   cultures (including gonorrhea and chlamydia).
7. Anticipate ultrasound examination (fill bladder).
8. Be prepared for other medical interventions
   appropriate for the problem the patient is
   experiencing.
9. If the patient did not receive $Rh_0(D)$ immune
   globulin and the blood work indicates that it is
   appropriate, administer in the E.D. if possible
   (see pp. 95–96).

Disposition and Instructions

If the patient is discharged home, her instructions should
include pelvic rest (nothing in vagina); follow-up with the

prenatal care provider (or give appropriate referrals); and instruction to seek immediate medical care for worsening of bleeding, cramping, or signs of infection.

ECTOPIC PREGNANCY

Description

An ectopic pregnancy is a pregnancy implanted anywhere other than the uterine cavity. Ninety-five percent of ectopic pregnancies occur in the fallopian tube (Cunningham et al., 1993). Other sites include the abdominal wall, the ovary, and the uterine ligaments. One percent of all reported pregnancies are ectopic, but ectopic pregnancy accounts for 6 to 7% of all maternal deaths, usually as a result of hemorrhage and shock (Cunningham et al., 1993).

Clinical and Diagnostic Findings

Signs and symptoms of pregnancy.
Abdominal and pelvic pain described as sudden, sharp, and stabbing occurs in 90%. In 20%, pain radiates to shoulder (intraperitoneal irritation).
Amenorrhea (average 5.5 weeks' duration) with vaginal spotting for 1 to 2 days.
Nausea with or without vomiting in 33%.
20% experience syncope.
66% have a pelvic mass.
20% present in shock out of proportion to the amount of vaginal bleeding observed.
Uterus enlarged in 16% because of the hormonal stimulation of pregnancy; may be displaced.
66% experience pain on cervical motion.
Exquisite tenderness and possible muscular rigidity on abdominal examination in 90%; rebound tenderness in 70%.
History may include history of previous ectopic pregnancy, pelvic inflammatory disease, infertility, endometriosis, intrauterine device use past or present, or tubal ligation (Jehle et al., 1994).
Serum qualitative hCG is positive in 89 to 100% 25 days after conception.
Quantitative hCG may be low for weeks' gestation.
WBC elevated (up to 15,000 in 50%).

Hemoglobin and hematocrit decreased depending on the degree of hemorrhage and may not yet correlate with an acute bleeding episode.

Differential Diagnoses

Differential diagnoses include pelvic inflammatory disease, abortion of intrauterine pregnancy, degenerating fibroids, ovarian cyst, gestational trophoblastic neoplasia, urinary tract infection, appendicitis, endometriosis, dysfunctional uterine bleeding, gastrointestinal disturbance, intrauterine pregnancy with another cause for pain, pelvic mass of another etiology, corpus luteum cyst, and ureteral calculi.

Nursing Actions

1. Maintain ABCs.
2. If patient is hemodynamically unstable, check pulse oximetry and administer supplemental oxygen if appropriate. Elevate the patient's legs.
3. Keep patient NPO.
4. Initiate large-bore intravenous line with lactated Ringer's and run at a rate appropriate for the patient's hemodynamic condition.
5. Draw blood for CBC, electrolytes, BUN, creatinine, hCG, PT, Ptt, type, Rh, and antibody screen (to determine the need for $Rh_0(D)$ immune globulin), and hold blood for crossmatching, sending for several units if the patient is hemodynamically unstable.
6. Send a clean-catch midstream sample for urinalysis; if suspicion is high for an ectopic pregnancy, place indwelling urinary catheter, send sample for urinalysis, and monitor output.
7. Anticipate gentle pelvic examination with cultures (including gonorrhea and chlamydia).
8. Anticipate ultrasound examination if the patient is hemodynamically stable (fill bladder).
9. Culdocentesis may be performed (see p. 104).
10. Explain procedures and findings to the patient and significant others.
11. Offer emotional support. If the patient is Catholic, offer to have the products of

conception baptized and arrange with the
surgical department.
12. Anticipate surgery for laparoscopy or
laparotomy, salpingectomy, or ipsilateral
oophorectomy (sterilization). If the pregnancy
is unruptured, anticipate salpingectomy,
segmental resection and anastomosis, or
evacuation of fimbriae.

FETAL DEMISE

Description

Fetal demise is intrauterine fetal death.

Clinical Signs and Diagnostic Findings May Include

Cessation of fetal movement.
Cessation of fetal growth or decreasing over time.
Absence of FHTs by fetoscope or Doppler.
Mother may report regression of symptoms of
pregnancy such as breast tenderness.
Mother may report recent weight loss.
Collapsed fetal skull noted on vaginal examination.
Ultrasound evidence of fetal death.
X-ray evidence of fetal death.

Nursing Actions

1. Take vital signs, including FHTs (see p. 6).
2. When FHTs cannot be found, assist with vaginal
   and abdominal examination and ultrasound or x-
   ray examinations.
3. Draw blood for CBC, PT, Ptt, platelets, fibrin
   split products, fibrinogen, peripheral smear, type,
   Rh, and antibody screen (to determine the need
   for $Rh_0(D)$ immune globulin).
4. Explain procedures and findings to the patient
   and her significant others.
5. Emotional support is extremely important for
   the patient. Allow significant others to be with
   the patient if possible. Offer to call a priest,

minister, or other spiritual adviser. The mother and her family will want to know why the baby has died. Avoid speculating about the cause of death but dispel myths concerning the cause of death such as the mother's having lifted a heavy object or having raised her hands over her head.

6. Anticipate the discussion of management options with the mother and her significant others. Labor can be induced, or expectant management would involve awaiting the onset of spontaneous labor. The risk of the latter is the development of disseminated intravascular coagulation. The patient is followed carefully with periodic laboratory studies (as listed previously) during the interval of waiting if this management option is chosen.

7. Should a woman give birth to a dead infant in the E.D., she, the baby's father, and other family members should be encouraged to view, touch, and hold the infant. Pictures may be taken and given to the parents—in a sealed envelope if desired. These interventions help ground the grieving process in reality and facilitate its resolution.

HYPERTENSION IN PREGNANCY

Description

Four categories of hypertension are associated with pregnancy: preeclampsia-eclampsia, chronic hypertension (of whatever etiology), preeclampsia-eclampsia superimposed on chronic hypertension, and transient hypertension. Preeclampsia-eclampsia is the disorder most often associated with severe maternal complications and posing the greatest danger to the fetus (Cunningham et al., 1993).

Preeclampsia complicates 6 to 8% of uterine pregnancies (Zuspan, 1991). It is a pregnancy-specific condition that usually occurs after 20 weeks' gestation, often near term, and sometimes in the first 24 hours postpartum. It is usually found in the primigravida or in a multigravida having her first child with a new partner (Fadigan et al., 1994). At increased risk are women at the age extremes of the childbearing years, women with twin pregnancies, severely obese women, women with chronic hypertension, and multiparous women with a history of previous preeclampsia (Stone et al., 1994).

The mother experiences widespread circulatory disturbances. She is at increased risk for abruptio placentae (21%), disseminated coagulopathy (8.3%), HELLP syndrome (see description following) (16.7%), acute renal failure (5%), pulmonary edema (5%), and eclampsia (16.7%) (Sibai, 1991). Eclampsia is severe preeclampsia with seizures caused by cerebral edema. When maternal death occurs, it is usually due to cerebral hemorrhage (Redman and Roberts, 1993).

The fetus suffers nutritional and respiratory deprivation because of suboptimal uteroplacental blood flow, is often small for gestational age, and may experience hypoxia and intrauterine death.

The HELLP syndrome (hemolysis, elevated liver enzymes, and low platelet count) is a variation of preeclampsia that is associated with a high maternal and perinatal mortality and morbidity. Patients usually present with epigastric or right upper quadrant pain and malaise and often with nausea and vomiting. Treatment is the same as for preeclampsia (Sibai, 1991).

Delivery usually causes rapid regression of the preeclampsia-eclampsia syndrome, with symptoms abating within 48 hours.

Clinical and Diagnostic Findings

Mild Preeclampsia

Edema—weight gain of 5 lb or more in a week; differentiate from dependent edema commonly seen in normal pregnancy; edema of the hands and particularly of the face is of concern.

Hypertension—an increase in the systolic blood pressure of 30 mm Hg or greater or an increase in diastolic blood pressure of 15 mm Hg or greater over the average value recorded before 20 weeks' gestation. If early readings are unknown, 140/90 after 20 weeks' gestation is considered positive.

Proteinuria—300 mg/24 hour urine collection or greater; 1+ protein in a random specimen (rule out other causes such as urinary tract infection).

Severe Preeclampsia

Hypertension—blood pressure 160 mm Hg or greater systolic or 110 mm Hg or greater diastolic on two occasions at least 6 hours apart with the patient at bed rest.

Proteinuria—5 g or greater per 24 hour urine collection or 3+ or greater on a dipstick in two random clean-catch samples at least 4 hours apart.

Oliguria.

Visual disturbances (scotoma, blurring, or other) or severe headache.

Epigastric pain.

Pulmonary edema.

Thrombocytopenia (<100,000 especially if the trend is downward) (Probst, 1994).

Serum creatinine greater than 1.2 mg/dL (if previously normal).

Increase in liver enzymes or jaundice.

Retinal hemorrhages, exudates, or papilledema.

HELLP Syndrome

Epigastric or right upper quadrant pain and malaise (90%).

Nausea and vomiting (50%).

Viral syndrome–like symptoms.

Hypertension may be absent in 20% and mild in 30%.

Hemolysis (abnormal peripheral smear, increased bilirubin ≥1.2 mg/dL, and increased lactate dehydrogenase [LDH]).

Elevated liver enzymes (serum aspartate aminotransferase [AST] ≥70 IU/I and elevated LDH).

Low platelet count (<100 × 10^3/mm^3) (Sibai, 1991).

Chronic Hypertension

Blood pressure 140/90 mm Hg or greater present before pregnancy or measured before 20 weeks' gestation (Probst, 1994).

Transient Hypertension

Development of hypertension during pregnancy or within 24 hours postpartum without signs and symptoms of preeclampsia or preexisting hypertension, returning to normal within 10 days postpartum (Probst, 1994).

Nursing Actions

1. Maintain ABCs.
2. Explain procedures and findings to the patient and her significant others. A calm and reassuring (although not falsely so) manner is particularly important with this patient.
3. Obtain vital signs, including FHTs, every 30 minutes or more.
4. Maintain complete bed rest. Position patient on her left side, lower the lights, minimize noise and stimulation, and employ seizure precautions.
5. Administer supplemental oxygen.
6. Initiate an intravenous line with a crystalloid fluid running no faster than 100 mL/hour.
7. Draw blood for CBC, electrolytes, serum creatinine, BUN, platelets, PT, Ptt, liver enzymes, and bilirubin.
8. Place indwelling urinary catheter. Dipstick urine for protein and send sample for urinalysis. Monitor output.
9. For the patient with persistent diastolic blood pressure greater than 100 mm Hg or signs of cerebral effects such as visual changes, severe headache, or hyperreflexia, anticipate the administration of $MgSO_4$ to prevent eclampsia (see p. 91) (Fadigan et al., 1994). Add the checking of deep tendon reflexes to the frequent vital signs.
10. Anticipate administration of antihypertensive medications for blood pressure greater than 110 mm Hg diastolic (see drug section, pp. 86–96).
11. Arrange for transfer to an obstetrical unit as soon as possible. At the obstetrical unit, fetal maturity and the maternal condition are weighed, and delivery is considered.

VAGINAL BLEEDING IN THE SECOND AND THIRD TRIMESTERS

Description

Possible causes of vaginal bleeding include placental abruption, placenta previa, or local cervical causes such as cervical polyps, cervical dysplasia, or cervicitis.

Note: A small amount of vaginal bleeding (often mucoid in nature) is often seen during labor at term as tiny capillaries are broken and bleed when the capillary-rich cervix effaces and dilates. This bleeding is self-limiting and accompanied by other signs of labor.

Placental Abruption

Description. Premature separation of part or all of a normally implanted placenta from the uterine wall causing maternal and fetal blood loss. The cause is unknown, but frequently associated factors include cigarette smoking, external trauma, pregnancy-induced or chronic hypertension, cocaine ingestion, uterine fibroids, preterm premature rupture of membranes, and a history of previous abruption (Cunningham et al., 1993).

Abruption occurs in 1 of every 200 deliveries and is fatal to the fetus in 1 of every 830 deliveries (Cunningham et al., 1993).

Clinical and Diagnostic Findings May Include

Labor may or may not be in progress.
Vaginal bleeding (may not be present if bleeding is
    encapsulated by still-attached placenta or
    membranes; Fig. 2–1).
Abdominal pain.
Tender, rigid, "board-like" uterus.
Irritable uterine activity.
Maternal hypovolemic shock may be present.
Mother may report decreased fetal movement.
Auscultation of FHTs may reveal nonreassuring
    pattern (see p. 6).
Hematocrit and hemoglobin may show anemia
    (unless bleeding was acute and recent).
Coagulation studies may show disseminated
    intravascular coagulation (decreased platelets,
    increased fibrin split products).
Ultrasound may confirm abruption but does not
    exclude it (confirmed only 25% in one study)
    (Cunningham et al., 1993).

Nursing Actions

1. Maintain ABCs.
2. **No vaginal examinations until placenta previa is ruled out.**

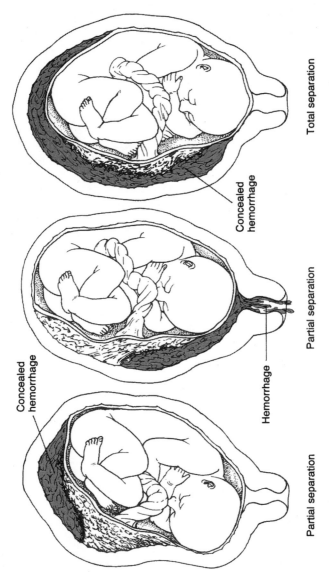

Figure 2–1. Placental abruption. Bleeding may be visible or concealed. (From Thompson, E. D. [1995]. Introduction to Maternity and Pediatric Nursing [2nd ed.]. Philadelphia: W. B. Saunders.)

3. Monitor vital signs including FHTs, every 15 minutes or more. Closely monitor blood loss. Remember that although the vital signs of a pregnant woman do not yet show decompensation, blood may be being shunted away from the uteroplacental bed, placing the fetus in grave danger from the maternal condition as well as from their own blood loss. Attend carefully to the woman's skin signs, mentation, and urine output as well as vital signs, and have a low threshold of suspicion for hypovolemia.

4. Position mother on her left side to displace the uterus off the inferior vena cava.

5. Administer supplemental oxygen.

6. Initiate large-bore intravenous line with lactated Ringer's and run at a rate appropriate for the patient's hemodynamic condition.

7. Draw blood for CBC, type, Rh, antibody screen (to determine need for $Rh_0(D)$ immune globulin), PT, Ptt, fibrinogen, fibrin split products, platelets, and a toxicology screen. Crossmatch a liberal number of units.

8. Blood should be given as quickly as possible to replace the oxygen-carrying capacity of the blood lost. Replace blood to a hematocrit of 30%, and give enough total fluids to maintain a urine output of 30 mL/hour. Observe the mother for signs of fluid overload, such as the presence of rales, coughing, or shortness of breath (Cunningham et al., 1993).

9. If hemodynamically unstable, place indwelling urinary catheter and monitor output closely. In any case, dipstick all urine for protein, send for urinalysis, and send for a toxicology screen.

10. Explain all procedures and findings to the patient and her significant others and offer emotional support.

11. If the fetus shows signs of severe compromise (persistent marked bradycardia or ominous decelerations; see p. 11), immediate cesarean section may be indicated. If the hospital has no obstetrical unit, consider whether a neonatal transport team could facilitate a safe delivery

or immediate transfer to a hospital with an obstetrical unit.
12. Transfer to an obstetrical unit.

Placenta Previa

Description. Site of placental implantation is located over or near the cervical os (Fig. 2–2). The placenta may be described as a total previa, a partial previa, or a marginal previa (with the edge of placenta at the margin of the cervical os). Placenta previa identified by ultrasound before the third trimester is a common finding because the proportion of placenta to uterine wall is great. In most cases, as the uterus grows, the placenta is said to "migrate" with the upper part of the uterus away from the cervical os, and the incidence at term is 1 in every 200 deliveries (Cunningham et al., 1993).

As pregnancy advances and the cervix undergoes the normal "ripening" in preparation for delivery, it thins and begins to open slightly. Blood vessels of the placenta are torn, and **painless** vaginal bleeding occurs. The bleeding is both maternal and fetal.

Clinical and Diagnostic Findings

Bright red painless vaginal bleeding.
Maternal shock may be present.
FHTs may demonstrate ominous patterns (see p. 11).
Fetus often in an abnormal position.
Ultrasound shows placenta over cervical os.
Hematocrit and hemoglobin may show anemia unless the blood loss has been acute and recent.

Nursing Actions

1. Maintain ABCs.
2. **No vaginal examinations** (neither speculum nor bimanual). Vaginal examination in the patient with placenta previa can cause **fatal hemorrhage** and can **only** be conducted in a delivery room with anesthesia, a scrubbed-in OR team, and a surgeon prepared to do an emergency cesarean section present (Cunningham et al., 1993).
3. Position mother on her left side to displace the uterus off the inferior vena cava.

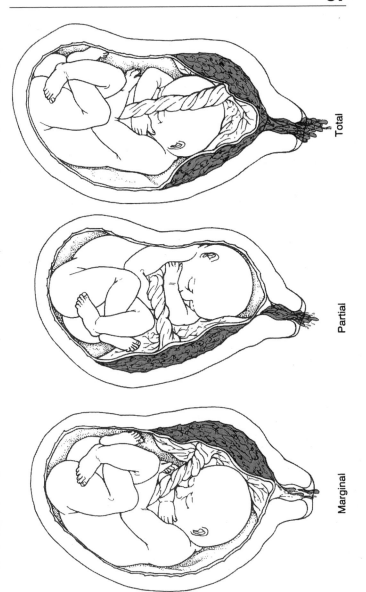

Figure 2–2. Placenta previa. (From Thompson, E. D. [1995]. Introduction to Maternity and Pediatric Nursing [2nd ed.]. Philadelphia: W. B. Saunders.)

4. Monitor vital signs of mother and FHTs every 15 minutes. Closely observe blood loss. Remember that although maternal vital signs do not yet show decompensation, blood flow may be being shunted away from the uteroplacental bed, and the fetus may be in grave danger because of the maternal condition as well as the fetus's own blood loss. Closely observe the mother's skin signs, mentation, and urine output and have a low level of suspicion for hypovolemia.

5. If the patient is hemodynamically unstable, administer supplemental oxygen.

6. Establish large-bore intravenous line with lactated Ringer's and run at a rate appropriate for the mother's hemodynamic condition.

7. Draw blood for CBC, clotting studies, type, Rh, and antibody screen (to determine need for $Rh_0(D)$ immune globulin).

8. If the patient is hemodynamically unstable, place indwelling urinary catheter and monitor output. In any case, send sample for urinalysis.

9. If obstetrical unit is in-house, transfer immediately.

10. Anticipate ultrasound examination. Fill bladder if indwelling urinary catheter not in place.

11. Explain all procedures and findings to the patient and her significant others and offer emotional support.

12. If the mother and fetus cannot be stabilized, immediate cesarean section is required. If the hospital is without an obstetrical department, consider the possibility of a neonatal transport team coming to the hospital to receive the neonate to facilitate a safe delivery, or transfer immediately to a hospital with an obstetrical department.

13. Arrange for transfer to an obstetrical unit for examination, monitoring, and possible cesarean section. If the bleeding has occurred before 37 weeks, the bleeding tapers, and mother and fetus are stable, the obstetrician may elect to continue the pregnancy with the mother hospitalized at bed rest (Cunningham et al.,

1993). In any case, cesarean section is the method of delivery.

SEXUALLY TRANSMITTED DISEASES IN PREGNANCY

Descriptions and Clinical and Diagnostic Findings

Acquired Immunodeficiency Syndrome (AIDS)

The incidence of AIDS among women of childbearing age in the United States is 0.015% (Martens, 1994). Transmission, which occurs by exchange of bodily fluids, occurs vertically (mother to fetus) prenatally, intrapartum (not improved by cesarean section), and postpartum (breast milk contains the virus). Risk of perinatal transmission is 25 to 35% (Martens, 1994). The latency period ranges from a few months to 10 years. The virus destroys the cells of the immune system. Studies have not consistently shown that AIDS influences pregnancy outcome. Antiviral agents have not been proven safe for the fetus. Diagnosis is made by testing serum for the presence of human immunodeficiency virus (HIV) by enzyme immunoassay (EIA), confirmed by the Western blot technique.

Herpes Simplex Virus (HSV)

Of the obstetrical population, 16.5% are seropositive for HSV, although only 0.5 to 1.0% demonstrate HSV by Pap smear or culture (Martens, 1994). Transmission occurs through sexual contact. The incubation period for the initial infection is 3 to 7 days. The disease is manifested by blister-like lesions, which shed the virus for 8 to 17 days. The initial outbreak may be accompanied by systemic symptoms, including fever, headaches, malaise, myalgia, nausea, and rarely meningitis and encephalitis. Lesions recur in 38 to 56%. Antivirals have not been proven safe in pregnancy. Herpes, particularly the initial outbreak, can cause spontaneous abortion, preterm labor, and intrauterine growth retardation. Neonatal herpes occurs in 1 of every 7500 births. Seventy percent are in infants whose mothers were unaware of an HSV history in themselves or their sexual partner. Intrauterine infection causes central nervous system anomalies. A woman with suspicious lesions at delivery should have the lesion cultured and should be delivered by cesarean section; appropriate specimens from the infant should be cultured (Cunningham et al., 1993). A woman with a positive history but no lesion at delivery can have a vaginal delivery and the infant observed.

The diagnosis of HSV infection is made by culture, Pap smear, and serological testing.

Syphilis

The incidence of congenital syphilis in the United States increased from 688 cases reported in 1988 to 2899 cases reported in 1990 (Chhabra et al., 1993). The incubation period is 10 to 90 days. Syphilis is manifested in stages: primary syphilis (a chancre, which may be small or located on the cervix and not noticed); secondary syphilis (a maculopapular rash frequently involving palms and soles with systemic symptoms and generalized lymphadenopathy); early latent syphilis (<1 year duration) (occasional exacerbations of mucocutaneous lesion); late latent syphilis (>1 year duration) (transmitted vertically but not sexually); and tertiary syphilis (central nervous system, cardiovascular, or musculoskeletal involvement).

Intrauterine infection causes spontaneous abortions, prematurity, stillbirth, and low birth weight, and the neonate exhibits involvement of the central nervous system, bone, blood, and kidney. Untreated, it causes abnormalities of facial bones and mouth, deafness, and mental retardation.

Diagnosis is made by a serological screening test, RPR or VDRL, which must be confirmed by a treponemal test, FTA-ABS or MHA-TP. The latter two tests remain positive permanently after infection.

Gonorrhea

The percentage of pregnant women in the United States who have gonorrhea is approximately 0.6 to 7.5% (Martens, 1994). One third of the neonates born to these women become infected at birth (Martens, 1994). Neonates show infection of the nasopharynx, the respiratory tract, the anal canal, and the eyes (ophthalmia neonatorum). Although symptoms can involve Skene's glands, Bartholin's glands, pharynx, vagina, and rectum, 75% of women are asymptomatic. The disease can become disseminated with fever, arthritis, cutaneous lesions, and endocarditis. During pregnancy, gonorrhea can cause spontaneous and septic abortions, endometritis, salpingitis, chorioamnionitis, premature rupture of membranes, preterm labor, and intrauterine growth retardation. At birth, ophthalmia neonatorum is prevented by giving all infants antibiotic eye prophylaxis within 1 hour of birth (Cunningham et al., 1993). After birth, puerperal sepsis in the mother can be caused by gonorrhea. Of patients who are positive for gonorrhea, 25 to 50% are also positive for chlamydia.

Diagnosis is made by culture.

Chlamydia trachomatis

The most common sexually transmitted disease (STD) in the United States, chlamydial infection affects about 5% of pregnant women in this country and up to 20% in impoverished or minority communities (Martens, 1994). The incubation period is 6 to 21 days, and it has a high coinfection rate with gonorrhea. Symptoms may be absent or minimal or may include cervicitis, bartholinitis, and acute ureteral syndrome; without treatment, pelvic inflammatory disease with sequelae of chronic pelvic pain, infertility, and ectopic pregnancy may occur. During pregnancy, chlamydial infection is associated with preterm labor, premature rupture of membranes, low birth weight, spontaneous abortion, and, rarely, pelvic inflammatory disease with 50% fetal wastage. Postpartum, endometritis is seen. Diagnosis is made by culture or antigen detection. To prevent chlamydial conjunctivitis, all infants receive antibiotic eye prophylaxis within 1 hour of birth (Cunningham et al., 1993).

Trichomonas

One of the most common STDs, *Trichomonas* was documented in 12.6% of women attending urban clinics in their midtrimester in one study (Martens, 1994). It commonly exists with other STDs, particularly gonorrhea and bacterial vaginosis. It is transmitted sexually, by fomites, and vertically. Vertical transmission occurs in 5% of pregnant women. Neonatal symptoms are purulent vaginitis, urinary tract infection, and pneumonia. Symptoms in the pregnant woman are an abnormal vaginal discharge, vulvar irritation, and, occasionally, abdominal pain.

Diagnosis is made by Pap smear, culture, and wet mount.

Bacterial Vaginosis

Bacterial vaginosis (previously called *Gardnerella* or *Haemophilus* infection) is a vaginal infection characterized by an overgrowth of anaerobic bacteria. It is transmitted sexually but not exclusively so. Bacterial vaginosis has been implicated in preterm labor, postpartum endometritis, and pelvic inflammatory disease. Forty percent of women are asymptomatic (Star, 1990). Others may complain of an unusual vaginal discharge that is gray, with a fishy odor, and vulvar irritation. Diagnosis is made by culture and wet mount. Concomitant STDs should be ruled out.

Nursing Actions

1. Take a sexual history: whether presently sexually active, number of recent partners, whether relationship is mutually monogamous, safe sex precautions used.
2. Anticipate gentle pelvic examination with cultures and wet mount. The patient who is suspected of having one STD should be tested for concurrent STDs.
3. Administer treatment as suggested in the Centers for Disease Control and Prevention Treatment Guidelines.
4. Provide emotional support to the patient to whom the occurrence of an STD and its implications are emotionally upsetting.
5. Report gonorrhea and syphilis to the local health department.

Discharge Instructions

1. Instruct the patient to have sexual partner(s) seek treatment.
2. Sexual abstinence is desirable until both partners have completed treatment. At the least, condoms should be used.
3. The patient who has contracted an STD sexually is not practicing safe sex and is at risk for all STDs, including HIV infection. Safe sex measures must be discussed, and the patient should be offered referral for HIV testing.

4. The patient should report the diagnosis and treatment to her prenatal health care provider for test-of-cure follow-up testing. If the patient is not receiving prenatal care, she should be given a referral.

TRAUMA DURING PREGNANCY

The pregnant trauma patient requires the same immediate emergency care as any other trauma patient: Maintain ABCs, immobilize the cervical spine, identify life-threatening chest injuries, and assess the level of consciousness (Sheehy et al. 1992). In addition, the pregnant trauma patient faces the following risks when experiencing trauma:

Placental abruption (see p. 33).
Rupture of membranes (see p. 71).
Premature labor (see p. 66).
Uterine laceration or rupture with fetal death.
Direct fetal injury (may be lethal even if maternal injuries are mild).
Extrauterine peritoneal bleeding.
Retroperitoneal hematoma.
Increased vulnerability to spleen, bowel, or bladder injury.
Amniotic fluid embolism.
Rh sensitization.
Engorged pelvic vasculature surrounding the pregnant uterus may be a significant source of bleeding with pelvic fractures.
Increased risk of maternal aspiration as a result of decreased gastric motility.

Special Considerations in Nursing Actions

1. *Quick action is vital for the pregnant patient who is still hemodynamically stable but is compensating for hypoperfusion.* There may be shunting of blood away from the uteroplacental unit, dangerously compromising the fetus. Therefore, the patient should be treated with a high level of suspicion for hidden hypoxia and hypoperfusion (Esposito, 1994).

2. If obstetrics is in-house, they should be called before or on arrival of the pregnant trauma patient to begin their assessment and interventions. In advanced pregnancy, a pediatrician should also be part of the team.
3. In any case of trauma, administer 100% supplemental oxygen because of increased oxygen consumption during pregnancy (Esposito, 1994).
4. Tilt or turn the patient to the left to prevent inferior vena cava compression and hypotension. An entire spinal board can be tilted with towels rolled under it.
5. In addition to the primary and secondary survey, assess the patient for uterine tenderness or contractions, vaginal bleeding, rupture of membranes, prolapse of umbilical cord, cervical dilation, and fetal movement.
6. When monitoring vital signs, remember FHTs (see p. 6). Remember that the pregnant woman's pulse is usually 10 to 15 bpm elevated and that the blood pressure is normally decreased by 5 to 15 mm Hg in midpregnancy.
7. Observe closely for signs and symptoms of hypovolemic shock, which may occur secondary to concealed hemorrhage.
8. In the case of hypovolemia, whole blood is infused as quickly as possible because of the extreme need for both mother and fetus to have fluids with oxygen-carrying capacity (Esposito, 1994).
9. The MAST suit may be used on the legs but **not** on the abdomen.
10. If fetomaternal bleeding is a concern (this may occur, for example, in placental abruption or uterine rupture), send a maternal blood specimen for a fetal hemoglobin or the Kleihauer-Betke examination by the laboratory, which examines maternal blood for the presence of fetal blood cells.
11. Ultrasound may be required to assess fetal condition.
12. Flat films of the abdomen are not helpful; computed tomography of the abdomen is suggested.

13. Whenever possible during x-ray examinations, shield the pregnant uterus with a lead apron.
14. Consider the emotional and spiritual needs of the woman whose fetus is in jeopardy as well as those of her significant others.
15. Consider the possible need for emergency cesarean section.
16. Tetanus toxoid may be given per usual protocols (Cefalo, 1996).
17. When stabilized, the pregnant trauma patient should be transferred to an obstetrical unit, where she and the fetus can be observed on an electronic fetal monitor for at least 24 to 48 hours.

URINARY TRACT INFECTION IN PREGNANCY

Special Considerations

1. The hormonal changes of pregnancy as well as the pressure on the bladder and urethra increase the pregnant woman's risk for developing urinary tract infection.
2. The symptoms of urinary tract infection may be masked by the hormonal milieu of pregnancy. Additionally, urinary frequency is already present in early and late pregnancy as a result of mechanical pressure on the bladder, and differentiation must be made. Of women who are asymptomatic but have bacteria in their urine, 20 to 30% go on to develop pyelonephritis if untreated (Abbott, 1994).
3. Pyelonephritis can precipitate premature labor (Abbott, 1994).
4. An important part of the management of the pregnant patient with a urinary tract infection is hydration.
5. If there is any question of premature labor (see p. 66 for complaints that may be signs of premature labor), the patient should be seen in an obstetrical unit for electronic fetal monitoring and obstetrical evaluation.

6. The patient should be instructed to contact her prenatal care provider immediately and arrange for a test-of-cure urine culture. If the patient is not receiving prenatal care, make this referral.

OVERDOSE AND SUBSTANCE ABUSE IN PREGNANCY

Special Considerations

1. Because of the immaturity of the fetal organs (particularly the liver), the drug(s) is present in the fetal system several times longer than it is in the mother's system.
2. The dose is far greater for the fetus than it is for the mother.
3. Anticipate transfer to an obstetrical unit for electronic fetal monitoring.
4. The teratogenic effects of any drug must be considered. Consult a toxicologist regarding the specific drug taken.
5. Refer for mental health follow-up.
6. Be certain that the prenatal care provider is aware of the overdose. The woman who intentionally overdoses during pregnancy is at high risk for postpartum depression. If she is not receiving prenatal care, give an appropriate referral.

RH INCOMPATIBILITY

Description

The Rh factor is an antigen present on the surface of red blood cells in the individual designated *Rh-positive.* Rh incompatibility occurs when the mother is Rh-negative and the fetus is Rh-positive. Rh sensitization, or Rh isoimmunization, occurs in this situation when fetal RBCs cross the placental barrier into the maternal circulation (see causes). The mother's immune system recognizes the Rh factor as foreign and produces IgG antibodies, which cross the placental barrier into fetal circulation and cause hemolysis of fetal RBCs (hemolytic disease of the newborn, or erythroblastosis fetalis). Sensitization is permanent, affecting all future pregnancies.

Events That May Cause Sensitization

Events that may cause sensitization include abdominal trauma, antenatal testing (chorionic villus sampling or amniocentesis), preterm labor, placental complications, any type of abortion, and ectopic pregnancy.

Prevention of Sensitization

$Rh_0(D)$ immune globulin, given as soon as possible and no more than 72 hours after any of the above-listed events, prevents Rh sensitization.

Nursing Actions

When any of the above-listed events has occurred to a pregnant woman, her blood type, Rh status, and antibody screen should be tested. If the woman has a positive antibody screen, she is already sensitized and $Rh_0(D)$ immune globulin is contraindicated (see pp. 95–96 regarding this medication).

CHAPTER THREE

Labor and Delivery

DESCRIPTION

Birth is a normal event that, ideally, is conducted with as little intervention as possible; the miracle of birth and the family are the focus. A birth that occurs in the emergency department (E.D.) is, however, in most cases, one for which the mother has had no prenatal care or one in which the labor has been precipitous and prenatal records are unavailable to emergency staff. Each of these situations presents risks for the mother and the fetus. Safeguards such as oxygen administration and intravenous access, therefore, are included in these guidelines for normal birth.

Although safety is the first concern, the staff should remember that birth is a life transition that will always be remembered by the family members and an event that may have a considerable effect on the self-esteem of the mother, who is very vulnerable at this time. Therefore, care should be given with special sensitivity to the emotional needs of the family. Keep the family together as much as possible. Provide privacy when possible. Your concern for their feelings and comfort will be meaningful for this family.

Birth is described as occurring in three stages:

First stage: From the onset of regular, effective contractions to complete dilation of the cervix (10 cm).

Second stage: From complete dilation of the cervix to delivery of the infant.

Third stage: From delivery of the infant to the delivery of the placenta and membranes.

FIRST STAGE OF LABOR

Clinical and Diagnostic Findings

Pregnancy is 37 to 42 weeks' gestation.

Uterine contractions may begin infrequently, at irregular intervals, or they can begin at an every-2-minute frequency (see palpation of uterine contractions, p. 11).

Amniotic membranes may be broken. The rupture may occur as a slow leak ("My underwear kept getting wet") or as a gush.

Some fetuses slow their movements as labor begins. Also, a distracted and uncomfortable mother may simply be less aware of fetal movement, but a complete cessation of fetal movement should not occur.

The *bloody show,* or the expelling of the mucus plug, occurs as the cervix begins effacement and dilation. This sign is considered a *soft sign* because it may occur weeks before, immediately before, or during labor.

The cervix dilates and effaces.

Nursing Actions

1. Transfer immediately to an in-house labor and delivery unit if there is one.
2. If possible, keep the patient's support person with her.
3. Check vital signs. The blood pressure should be checked with the patient on her left side between contractions. Fetal heart tones should be checked as described on page 6 every 15 minutes.
4. Ask the woman for a brief obstetrical history, especially the size of her largest previous baby (a larger baby poses the danger of shoulder dystocia); the length of her last labor (to help in deciding whether she can be transferred before delivery); whether she has had a cesarean section and, if so, whether her uterus was cut in the transverse or vertical direction (not necessarily the same direction as the visible scar; vaginal birth is contraindicated following a vertical incision); whether she hemorrhaged after the birth (increasing the risk of postpartum hemorrhage with this birth); or any other complications of pregnancy, birth, or postpartum.
5. Ask the woman for a brief history of the present pregnancy: EDC; whether she received

prenatal care; and complications, especially vaginal bleeding (placenta previa contraindicates vaginal delivery), gestational diabetes (neonate should be observed closely after delivery for hypoglycemia), malposition, hypertension, or herpes (a current lesion contraindicates vaginal delivery).

6. Ask the woman for a labor history: onset of contractions; frequency, length, and strength of contractions (can you walk or talk through them?); rupture of membranes (either a slow leak or a gush) and if so when and color of fluid; whether the baby is moving; and whether any drugs have been ingested.

7. Note whether there is dependent edema. Check deep tendon reflexes and clonus (assessing for preeclampsia).

8. Time and palpate uterine contractions (see pp. 11 and 12).

9. If membranes are grossly ruptured, test with Nitrazine paper (to rule out urinary incontinence) and document. If a slowly leaking rupture of membranes is suspected, assist with a sterile speculum examination (see p. 110). Time of rupture and color of fluid should be noted. FHTs should be checked immediately on rupture, and a digital vaginal examination should be done to rule out a prolapsed umbilical cord (see p. 75) and to assess progress in labor (see p. 16).

10. If delivery is imminent (see p. 52), a manual vaginal examination should be done to assess progress in labor (see pp. 13 and 14).

11. Obtain a clean-catch urine specimen and dipstick for protein. Amniotic fluid, blood, and cervical mucus cause a false-positive result. The woman should be catheterized with a nonindwelling catheter for a specimen only if there is a strong suspicion of preeclampsia.

12. Establish a large-bore intravenous line with lactated Ringer's solution.

13. Draw blood for CBC, type, Rh, antibody screen (to determine the need for $Rh_0(D)$

immune globulin), VDRL or RPR, and a toxicology screen if indicated.
14. Administer supplemental oxygen.
15. Keep the mother in a left side-lying position.
16. Provide the woman with any possible comfort measures (e.g., cool cloth to forehead, pillows behind back and between knees).
17. Explain all procedures, findings, and management plan to patient and her significant others.
18. If there is no in-house obstetrical unit and if delivery does not appear to be imminent (see next section), arrange for emergency transport to an obstetrical unit.
19. If delivery is imminent, prepare for delivery.

SECOND STAGE OF LABOR

Signs of Imminent Delivery

1. Contractions are most often occurring every 2 to 3 minutes.
2. The woman makes involuntary grunting sounds.
3. The perineum bulges, a bloody/mucoid discharge may be present, and the presenting part may be seen.
4. The patient tells you the baby is coming.
5. The FHTs may drop in rate during second-stage contractions. Known as an "early deceleration," this vagal response to pressure on the head is not dangerous *as long as* the rate springs back to the baseline *as soon* as the contraction is over, and the rate stays above 100 (Gabbe et al., 1991).

Preparation for Delivery

1. Place mother in left side-lying position.
2. Administer supplemental oxygen by nasal cannula.
3. If not in place, initiate large-bore intravenous line with lactated Ringer's solution.
4. If not done, draw blood for CBC, Rh, type, antibody screen (to determine need for $Rh_0(D)$ immune globulin), VDRL, and toxicology screen if indicated.

5. Assist the patient to empty her bladder (a safety measure for postpartum hemorrhage). Use nonindwelling urinary catheter if necessary. Dipstick for protein and send sample for urinalysis.
6. Reassure the patient, and make her as comfortable as possible. If possible, allow support person to stay with the mother.
7. Repeat maternal blood pressure, pulse, and respiration every 30 minutes.
8. Ideally, listen to FHTs after every contraction. At the least, listen every 5 minutes. Remember, the fetus is moving down the birth canal and FHTs will be auscultated lower and lower on the abdomen.

Equipment and Instruments

1. Turn isolette on to 37°C.
2. Set up oxygen in isolette.
3. Get several warm blankets from the blanket warmer. Keep them in the isolette, which is warming.
4. Open the delivery pack.
5. Prepare suction.
6. Draw up oxytocin (Pitocin) 10 units in each of two syringes, labeling each, so that they can be given readily after delivery.
7. Set out tubes for fetal bloodwork (to be collected from the placental side of the umbilical cord after delivery or drawn from placental vessels). Blood samples for CBC, VDRL, type and Rh, and Coombs' test should be sent. If there is concern about maternal drug use, add a drug screen.
8. Have several blankets or pillows on standby so that if the delivery occurs with the woman on her back, she can be tilted to her left side to avoid inferior vena cava compression.

Conduct of Delivery

1. Assist the mother into a position of comfort with the **uterus tilted to the left off the inferior**

vena cava. Someone should be stationed at her sides (support people can do this) to support her legs as she pushes with each contraction (instead of using stirrups). By palpating the uterus and speaking in low tones to the mother, help her push with the contractions by following her body's urges. She should **rest between contractions.**

2. **Once the head is actually emerging, coach the mother to blow through the contractions**—"like blowing out a birthday candle" or "pant like a puppy dog." The uterus itself delivers the baby, the more slowly, the more controlled. If the bag of waters is still intact, the deliverer uses the Kelly clamp and breaks it now. Note the color of the fluid—a green or yellow tint is meconium (see p. 72).

3. Using the palm of the hand, the deliverer should simply **apply steady counterpressure as the head emerges,** so that it emerges as slowly as possible.

4. Once the head is delivered, **firmly coach the mother to blow** (and not push—a very difficult request) while the deliverer **thoroughly suctions the mouth and then the nose** (stimulation of the nose may cause respiration before the mouth contents have been suctioned). **If the fluid is meconium stained, this step is extremely important.**

5. The deliverer **feels around the baby's neck for the umbilical cord.** If it is there, the loop is pulled around the head. If it is too short for that, two Kelly clamps are used to clamp the cord twice, and the cord is cut between the two Kellys and unwrapped from the neck.

   Alternatively, the baby can be delivered through the loop of cord.

6. The baby's body is supported as it emerges. The anterior shoulder and then the posterior shoulder deliver. For difficulty with the delivery of the shoulders, see page 76. The inexperienced deliverer should allow the woman's body to turn the baby as necessary and should not risk maneuvering and injuring the baby. The baby's body is delivered upward as though to lay it on

the mother's belly as it emerges (this brings the baby along the natural curve of the birth canal). The baby is kept near the level of the uterus to prevent a transfusion from infant to placenta or vice versa (Fig. 3–1).

7. The cord is clamped and cut, if it was not done previously, at least 6 inches from the umbilical stump. **Lay the baby directly on the mother's stomach skin to skin and cover with a warm blanket.** The mother's body is an excellent incubator. Immediately dry the infant and cover again with dry warm blankets. (**If the infant does not respond and begin breathing, see p. 62.**)

8. Note infant's birth time.

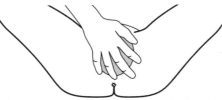

A Apply steady counterpressure as the head emerges.

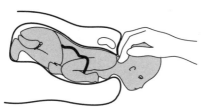

B Feel for the umbilical cord at the neck.

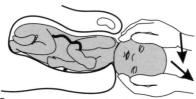

C Delivery of the anterior shoulder.

Figure 3–1. Conduct of delivery.
Illustration continued on following page

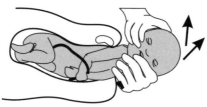

D Delivery of the posterior shoulder.

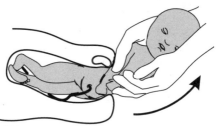

E Delivery of body following the
natural curve of the birth canal.

Figure 3–1. *Continued*

THIRD STAGE OF LABOR

Until the Placenta Is Ready to Deliver

1. **Never turn your back on the perineum.**
   Someone **must** be assigned to observe the
   perineum for bleeding and for signs of placental
   separation. Lethal hemorrhage can occur in
   minutes during the third stage.
2. For bleeding from perineal lacerations or an
   episiotomy, use gauze and apply pressure.
3. Remember that greater than 500 mL blood loss
   is defined as a postpartum hemorrhage. If this
   occurs, see page 82 regarding postpartum
   hemorrhage.
4. The following three signs indicate that the
   placenta is separating and may be ready for
   delivery:
   Lengthening of the cord.
   A small gush of bleeding.
   A rising up of the uterus as the placenta drops out.

Usually the woman experiences a uterine contraction at this time, and she may complain of a backache, pelvic pressure, or the urge to push.

Normal Length of Third Stage

Greater than 1 hour is considered *prolonged* third stage. Greater than 2 hours is considered "*maximum.*" These limits are for controlled circumstances (i.e., labor and delivery). In the absence of hemorrhage, risks and benefits must be weighed before intervening.

When the Placenta Has Separated

1. The third stage of labor carries dangerous risks for the mother and requires skill on the part of the birth assistant. It is most desirable to have a skilled birth assistant conducting this stage. As long as vaginal bleeding is minimal, delivery of the placenta can await the arrival of a transport delivery team.

2. One of the deliverer's hands should be placed just above the symphysis pubis, preventing the uterus from being pulled out and inverting with the delivery of the placenta. With the second hand, the birth assistant should apply steady downward pressure on the clamp on the umbilical cord. If the placenta does not move steadily down, further signs of placental separation are awaited. If the placenta does come, just as it appears at the introitus, the cord is lifted upward so that the placenta is following the curve of the birth canal as it delivers. The placenta is delivered into the basin from the instrument table.

3. If the mother has an urge to push, an excellent alternative to the aforementioned delivery technique is to assist the mother to a squatting position (with someone on each arm) and allow her to push the placenta out. This decreases the risk of attempting delivery before the placenta is fully separated and thus inverting the uterus—a lethal complication.

4. **Note time of placental delivery** and whether it delivered dull or shiny side up.

After Delivery of the Placenta

1. Hemostasis must be established by full contraction of the uterus: **Run intravenous line with 10 to 40 units Pitocin wide open. Massage the uterus firmly** (this is uncomfortable for the mother—you are rubbing a sore muscle). If bleeding is not easily controlled, see Postpartum Hemorrhage, page 82.
2. Repair of the perineum should be undertaken *only* to establish hemostasis (if pressure application fails to do so) or by an experienced birth assistant.
3. The placenta should be inspected for completeness and for normalcy.
4. The placenta is filled with the baby's blood. Fill the following tubes with this fetal blood, if not collected earlier: two plain red tops, a purple, and another plain red top if a toxicology screen is indicated. The blood can be collected from the cut cord by opening the clamp, milking the blood out of the cord if necessary. If more is needed, turn the placenta shiny side up and draw with a needle and syringe from the large vessels easily visible. Double-bag the placenta, and transfer it and the fetal bloods to the receiving hospital with the mother.

THE FIRST POSTPARTUM HOUR

Care of the Mother

1. Check **vital signs** every 15 minutes for four times then every hour for four times.
2. Every 15 minutes, or more frequently if the patient is not stable, **firmly massage the uterus** and note the amount of bleeding from the perineum. The uterus should be centrally located 1 to 2 fingerbreadths under the umbilicus. It should feel rock-hard. It may feel boggy and require firm massage to expel clots

before it feels rock-hard. Normally, in the first hour, the bleeding saturates approximately one peripad every 15 minutes.

3. Make the mother comfortable. Apply two peripads and a fresh underpad so that the amount of vaginal bleeding is easily seen.

4. Apply an ice bag to the perineum.

5. **Keep the bladder empty.** The patient should be offered the bedpan. A full bladder prevents uterine contraction and increases bleeding. If the patient is bleeding heavily, if the uterus is shifted to either side, or if the bladder is distended and the patient cannot void, do a straight catheterization to empty the bladder, thereby allowing stabilization of the bleeding.

6. If the vaginal bleeding is heavy, see Postpartum Hemorrhage, page 82. Maintain the intravenous line with 10 to 40 units of Pitocin per liter of crystalloid solution running rapidly for the first liter, scaling back to 125 to 200 mL/hour with subsequent liters if bleeding is stabilized.

7. If the patient is hypertensive, the left side remains the position of choice. The uterus is still large enough to compress the inferior vena cava.

8. Remain alert for signs of preeclampsia, which can manifest in the first 24 hours postpartum (see p. 29).

9. Remember the emotional aspects of the first postpartum hour, which many believe is crucial in the **bonding** process. Allow the mother to hold the baby or her support person to hold the baby at her side. Remember that the more stressed the mother, the more the mother-infant relationship will benefit from whatever bonding time and positive affirmations you can offer the mother. Involve the significant others to whatever extent possible.

10. If the mother plans to breast-feed, assist her to do so.

Follow-up

Mothers often go over and over the details of their deliveries, particularly if the labor was tumultuous and there was a lot happening that could not be explained at the time, or if the mother was in advanced labor and unable to take in all the events. A call or visit and a review of the birth may be an important therapeutic intervention. The new mother is particularly emotionally vulnerable and will be appreciative that you cared enough about her to follow up.

Immediate Care of the Newborn

Basic Principles

Keep baby warm.
Support transition to life (breathing).
Maintain blood glucose.

Nursing Actions

1. Gently dry the baby in a warm blanket, then wrap the baby snugly in another dry warm blanket. Remember to cover the baby's head as well. If the baby is placed in a prewarmed isolette, dry the infant, but do not cover it so that the radiant heat reaches the baby. This accomplishes two things: The baby is kept warm and is gently stimulated to begin breathing.
2. Observe the baby's initial respiratory efforts. Suction gently (use bulb, or wall suction at 60 to 80 mm Hg). Some babies begin with a gasp and a cry; others simply slowly start to breathe. The normal rate is 30 to 60 respirations/minute. The infant may do both diaphragmatic and abdominal breathing. Infants are obligate nose-breathers. Signs of respiratory distress include grunting, flaring nares, intercostal and xiphoid retractions, and a low rate or absence of respirations.
3. Auscultate the baby's heart rate. The normal rate is 120 to 160. A rate below 100 requires intervention (see p. 62).
4. Observe the baby for a gradual improvement in the color of the trunk. The healthy newborn's extremities often remain blue, but cyanosis of the trunk requires intervention (see p. 62).

5. Note the Apgar score at 1 and 5 minutes (Table 3–1). **Do not delay resuscitation to assign Apgar score.** Score infant at 1 and 5 minutes and at 5-minute intervals while resuscitating. Severity of Apgar scores:

   8–10 normal; no asphyxia
   5–7 mild asphyxia
   3–5 moderate asphyxia
   0–2 severe asphyxia

   A baby in distress deteriorates in the following order: color and respiratory status deteriorate, heart rate slows, muscle tone diminishes, and reflexes cease. Factors that can affect the Apgar score include hypoxia, prematurity, maternal sedation or analgesia, muscular diseases, and cerebral malformations.

6. Leave the umbilical cord at least 6 inches long. This can always be trimmed later but may be used by the neonatologist at the receiving hospital to establish venous access.

7. Observe baby for **jitteriness** or other signs of hypoglycemia (apathy; abnormal cry; hypothermia; irregular respirations; and ultimately apnea, cyanosis, tremors, limpness, and convulsions) (Varney, 1987). If these signs occur or if the baby is at risk for hypoglycemia (premature; small for gestational age; diabetic mother; asphyxiation, cold stress, or congenital defect), check the blood glucose by performing

Table 3–1. Apgar Score

Characteristic	Score		
	0	**1**	**2**
Color	Blue or pale	Trunk pink, extremities blue	Pink all over
Respiratory effort	Absent	Slow, irregular weak cry	Crying lustily
Heart rate	Absent	<100	>100
Muscle tone	Limp	Some flexion of limbs	Active movement
Reflexes	Absent	Facial grimace	Crying

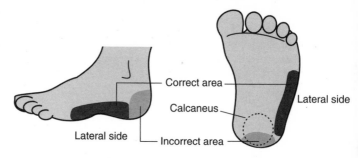

Figure 3–2. Appropriate area for heelstick.

a heelstick (Fig. 3–2), using a Dextrostix or the equivalent. If the reading is less than 60 and the mother wants to breast-feed, encourage the mother to do so at this time. If the mother wants to bottle-feed, have her give the baby dextrose water. Recheck the blood glucose in 20 minutes (Table 3–2).

8. Maintain the infant's body temperature with fresh warm blankets. Check the temperature every 30 minutes for the first hour to make sure the baby is maintaining a normal temperature (35 to 37°C axillary).

9. Administer vitamin K into the baby's thigh (see p. 97).

10. After the family has had time together, and after the mother has had an opportunity to breast-feed the baby (but within 1 hour of birth) (Martens, 1994), administer erythromycin eye ointment (see p. 88).

Neonatal Resuscitation

1. Gently **dry** infant and place in a warmed isolette in the **"sniff" position** (neck slightly extended; see Fig. 3–3) in a slight Trendelenburg position. A ¾ to 1 inch roll under the baby's shoulders helps to maintain this position.

2. Throughout the interventions, **keep infant warm.** Cold stress alone can delay recovery from acidosis (Chameides and Hazinski, 1994).

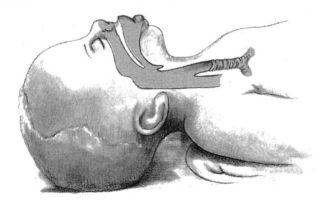

Figure 3–3. Sniff position for neonatal resuscitation. *Note:* A small towel under the shoulders assists in maintaining the slight hyperextension of the head. (From Gorrie, T. M. [1994]. Foundations of Maternal Newborn Nursing. Philadelphia: W. B. Saunders, p. 841.)

3. Provide **gentle stimulation** (gently rub back or flick heels).
4. If respiratory rate is good and pulse is greater than 100 but **trunk is cyanotic, administer** 10 L warm and humidified **oxygen** by holding a mask near the infant's face.
5. If **respiratory distress** is evident (irregular or absent efforts, grunting, flaring, retractions), administer **positive pressure ventilation** with 100% oxygen with a bag-mask–valve that delivers 20 to 30 cm H_2O pressure, with a bypassable popoff valve and an oxygen reservoir. The first breath may require up to 40 to 50 cm H_2O pressure; thereafter, use 20 to 30 cm H_2O pressure. Begin slowly and observe volume and force necessary for adequate chest expansion to avoid pneumothorax. Deliver a puff every 1 to 2 seconds (rate 30 to 60). If bag-mask–valve ventilation is still necessary after 2 minutes, pass an 8-Fr feeding tube down the mouth to decompress the stomach.
6. If the heart rate remains 100 after 30 seconds of adequate ventilation, **begin chest compressions** using two thumbs on the lower one third of the sternum encircling the body or using the third

Table 3-2. Normal Neonatal Laboratory Values

	From Cord Blood	Fingerstick	Venous
RBC	3.9–5.5/mm³	at 1–3 days 4.0–6.6/mm³	at 2 weeks 3.6–6.2/mm
Hct		1st day 48–69%	3rd day 44–72%
Hgb		at 1–3 days 14.5–22.5 g/100 mL	
WBC			at birth 9.0–30.0/mm 24 hours 9.4–34.0/mm 1 month 5.0–19.5/mm
Platelets			200,000–500,000

Differential
bands	3–5
segs	54–62
lymphs	25–33
monos	3–7
eos	1–3
basos	0–0.75

Urinalysis
RBCs	0
WBCs	0
epithelial cells	few
tubular epithelium	0
protein	neg
glucose	neg
ketones	neg
bilirubin	neg
specific gravity	1.002–1.015

Coombs' (indirect or direct) negative

Glucose
50–60 mg/100 mL	normal
40 mg/100 mL	suspect hypoglycemia
30 mg/100 mL	increased concern
20 mg/100 mL	treat for hypoglycemia

Arterial Blood Gases

	Birth	1 hour	24 hours
pH	7.26	7.30	7.40
P_{CO_2}	54.5	38.8	33.6
P_{O_2}	<55	60	90
HCO_3	24	21	21

Serum Bilirubin

cord	<2.0 mg/dL
0–1 day	<6.0 mg/dL
0–2 days	<8.0 mg/dL
2–5 days	<12.0 mg/dL
later	0.2–1.0 mg/dL

The highest the bilirubin should normally go is birth weight divided by 100 (e.g., for the 2500 g baby, 25 g/dL)
>20 mg/dL or a rise of 0.5 mg/dL in 1 hour requires an exchange transfusion
>15 mg/dL requires phototherapy

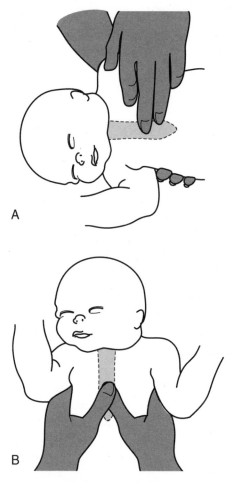

A

B

Figure 3–4. *A* and *B*, Chest compressions for neonatal resuscitation. Finger placement is on the lower third of the sternum, above the xiphoid process. The compression depth is ½ to ¾ inch. The rate is 120 bpm with a respiration interspersed every third beat. Compression is smooth, with the compression phase equaling the relaxation phase.

Table 3–3. Medications Used for Neonatal Resuscitation

Medication and Concentration	Dose and Route	Precautions
Epinephrine, 1 : 10,000	0.01–0.03 mg/kg IV or ET (equals 0.1–0.3 mL/kg)	Give rapidly; repeat every 3–5 minutes
Volume expanders (5% albumin, blood, normal saline, Ringer's lactate)	10 mL/kg IV	Reassess after each bolus
Naloxone, 0.4 mg/mL or 1.0 mg/mL	0.1 mg/kg IV, ET, SQ, IM	Give rapidly; repeat every 2–3 minutes
Bicarbonate 8.4% (1.0 mEq/mL) solution diluted 1 : 1 with sterile water to reduce hypertonicity	1–2 mEq/kg (equals 2–4 mL/kg)	**Ensure adequate ventilation first; useful only in prolonged resuscitation for ABG-documented acidosis**

IM = Intramuscular; ET = endotracheal; SQ = subcutaneous; IV = intravenous, including intraosseous.

Note: Drugs given endotracheally are followed with 0.5 mL sterile water to flush the tube.

Adapted from Chameides, L., and Hazinski, M. F. (Eds.) (1994). Textbook of Pediatric Advanced Life Support. Dallas: American Heart Association and American Academy of Pediatrics. Reproduced by permission. *Textbook of Pediatric Life Support,* 1994. © Copyright American Heart Association.

and fourth fingers on the lower one third of the sternum (Fig. 3–4). **Compress ½ to ¾ inch 120 times a minute, interspersing a breath every third beat.** Compressions should be smooth, and the compression phase should equal the relaxation phase.

7. If spontaneous respirations do not occur after bagging the infant, an individual trained in neonatal intubation should **intubate** the infant. A chest x-ray should be taken to confirm placement.

8. **Medications** are given as noted in Table 3–3. The Broselow Resuscitation Tape is a length-based resuscitation tape that gives an estimate of weight, equipment sizes, and drug doses for infants over 3 kg. A resuscitation tape for full-term and premature newborns is also being developed

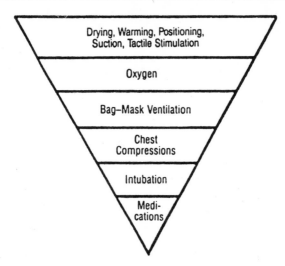

Figure 3–5. Inverted pyramid reflecting the approximate relative frequencies of neonatal resuscitation measures. (From the American Heart Association and the American Academy of Pediatrics. [1994]. Pediatric Advanced Life Support. Dallas: American Heart Association.)

(Khan and Luten, 1994). The endotracheal tube can be used as a route for medications as noted in Table 3–3. Use a 5-Fr feeding tube to instill the drug and flush with 0.5 mL respiratory sterile normal saline. Drugs may also be given into an umbilical catheter or by intraosseous, intramuscular, or subcutaneous routes.

Figure 3–5 illustrates the approximate relative frequencies of neonatal resuscitation measures.

COMPLICATIONS OF LABOR AND DELIVERY

Premature Labor

Description

Premature labor is defined as uterine contractions with cervical effacement and dilation before 37 weeks' gestation. Premature labor complicates 8 to 10% of all pregnancies (Gianopoulos, 1994). Infection, although often silent, is presumed to be the most common cause of preterm labor.

Clinical and Diagnostic Findings May Include

Abdominal "tightness," "pressure," "cramps," or
  pain.
Back discomfort.
Pelvic pressure.
Discomfort may or may not be rhythmic.
Increased frequency of bowel movements.
Leaking of fluid from vagina.
Increased vaginal secretions.
Bloody or mucoid vaginal discharge.
Amniotic membranes may be ruptured (see p. 110).
Cervix is changed from closed, posterior, and firm.
Presenting part is low in the pelvis.

▶ NOTE: *Premature labor can be manifested subtly and
  such signs should be taken seriously. See page 71 for
  discussion of preterm rupture of membranes, which may occur
  simultaneously.*

Differential Diagnoses

Differential diagnoses include normal fetal activity, gastrointestinal activity, irritability of uterus caused by dehydration, preterm rupture of membranes without labor (see p. 71), urinary tract infection, vaginitis, cervicitis, chorioamnionitis, and Braxton Hicks contractions (normal uterine activity).

Nursing Actions

1. If labor and delivery is in-house, transfer
   immediately.
2. Time several of the sensations the patient is
   describing, palpating the uterus as described on
   pages 11 and 12.
3. Take vital signs, including FHTs (see p. 6).
4. If ruptured membranes are suspected, a sterile
   speculum examination should be done (see p.
   110). Cultures should be carried out to detect
   infection, including gonorrhea, chlamydial
   infection, and beta streptococcal infection.
   Cervical effacement and dilation should be
   visually estimated. Note whether the umbilical
   cord can be visualized (see p. 75). Note the
   color of fluid if it is present.

5. If the membranes are ruptured, every cervical examination increases the risk of chorioamnionitis, which may shorten the time the pregnancy can continue. A few days might be vital for an immature infant. If labor is active and the decision whether to transfer now or after delivery depends on knowing the precise cervical dilation, a manual examination has to be done. If the FHTs are not reassuring (see p. 9), a manual examination must be done to rule out umbilical cord prolapse. If labor is not active, however, and FHTs are reassuring, a manual vaginal examination should not be done. (See p. 71 for further discussion of the management of the patient with preterm rupture of membranes.)

6. Once ruptured membranes have been ruled out, a *gentle* manual examination of the cervix can be done.

7. Initiate an intravenous line with crystalloid fluids. A bolus of 500 mL may be ordered to see if contractions stop with rehydration.

8. Anticipate assessment for possible causative factors: urinary tract infection (see p. 45), preeclampsia (see p. 29), maternal fever or sepsis, drug ingestion (particularly cocaine) (see p. 46), maternal autoimmune disease, maternal diabetes, placental abruption (see p. 33), placenta previa (see p. 36), trauma (see p. 43), or complications of the present pregnancy (e.g., multiple fetuses, fibroids, or fetal abnormalities) (Gianopoulos, 1994). An obstetrical history should be taken, including risk factors (history of premature labor, placental insufficiency, small-for-dates baby, familial congenital syndromes).

9. If contractions persist, anticipate the administration of magnesium sulfate (see p. 91) or terbutaline (see p. 96).

10. Arrange for transfer to an obstetrical unit. The aforementioned complaints are not thoroughly investigated until the patient has been evaluated on the electronic fetal monitor by a certified nurse-midwife or an obstetrician.

Preterm Rupture of Membranes

Description

Preterm rupture of membranes is rupture of amniotic membranes before 37 weeks' gestation, 2 hours or more before the onset of labor (Gianopoulos, 1994). The main maternal complication is chorioamnionitis. Before 26 weeks, the fetal death rate is 15%, and the neonatal death rate is 39% (Ghidini and Romero, 1994). Gestational age at delivery determines the outcome (Ghidini and Romero, 1994). Preterm rupture of membranes occurs in 1.7% of pregnancies (Cunningham et al., 1993). Most of these patients are in labor within 48 hours.

Complications from preterm rupture of membranes are amnionitis, endometritis, prematurity, respiratory distress syndrome, asphyxia, malpresentation, cord prolapse, cord compression, and fetal injuries secondary to low amniotic fluid volume. The occurrence of chorioamnionitis is directly proportional to the number of vaginal examinations (Gianopoulos, 1994).

Clinical and Laboratory Findings

Patient reports fluid coming from the vagina.
Fever, chills, and a malodorous discharge may
  indicate infection.

Differential and Concurrent Diagnoses

Other possible diagnoses include preterm labor, amnionitis, umbilical prolapse, incontinence, vaginal secretions, and fetal demise.

Nursing Actions

1. If labor and delivery is in-house, transfer
   immediately.
2. Take vital signs, including FHTs. The presence
   of fever is significant in preterm rupture of
   membranes.
3. A sterile speculum examination should be done.
   Cultures, including for gonorrhea, *C. trachomatis,*
   and beta streptococcus, should be obtained.
   Cervical effacement and dilation should be

visually estimated. The examiner should note whether the umbilical cord can be visualized (see p. 75). The color of the fluid should be noted.

4. Question the mother about back, abdominal, or pelvic discomfort, which might indicate labor.
5. If the membranes are ruptured, every cervical examination increases the risk of chorioamnionitis, which may shorten the time the pregnancy can continue. If the woman is not contracting actively, and if FHTs are reassuring, digital examination should be deferred.
6. If there is fetal distress, vaginal examination is indicated to rule out umbilical cord prolapse and to measure progress in labor to make a transfer plan.
7. Initiate intravenous line with crystalloid fluid. A 500-mL bolus may be ordered to attempt to slow down uterine activity with rehydration.
8. Arrange for transfer to a hospital with an obstetrical unit. If delivery is imminent, consider calling a neonatal transfer team to come to your E.D.
9. Expectant management is usually the plan for preterm rupture of membranes before 33 weeks. At the receiving hospital, tocolytics may be used to prolong the pregnancy and corticosteroids may be given to hasten lung maturity (Cunningham et al., 1993). If the pregnancy is 33 weeks or more, induction is generally the management plan (Cunningham et al., 1993).

Meconium

Description

Meconium is fetal stool that is passed either in the course of normal maturation (especially in the postdates fetus) or during a hypoxic period that caused the anal sphincter to relax. Whether the hypoxia was transient or whether it is continuing cannot be proven; therefore, fetal hypoxia must be assumed. The degree of meconium staining is described as "1+" or "light" (fluid is lightly tinted yellow or green); "3+" (opaque and thick, with particulate matter, described as "pea soup"); and 2+, which is somewhere between.

Dangers

1. The fetus may be compromised in utero and may require resuscitation at birth.
2. If meconium is aspirated with the first breath, a potentially fatal pneumonia may develop.

Nursing Actions

1. When meconium is identified with the rupture of membranes, the urgency of transferring the mother to deliver in a hospital with a neonatal intensive care unit is increased. Alternatively, consider calling a neonatal transport team to come to your hospital to assist in resuscitating and then transporting the infant.
2. Position the mother on her left side.
3. Administer supplemental oxygen.
4. Initiate a large-bore intravenous line with crystalloid fluid and administer rapidly.
5. Have someone at the delivery who is skilled in neonatal intubation.
6. Prepare the intubation equipment, suction, oxygen, and a warm area for the intubation of the infant.
7. Prepare a suction catheter at the delivery area for suction at birth.
8. Instruct the mother that once the head is delivered, it is crucial for her to blow and not push (like blowing out a birthday candle or panting like a puppy). This is difficult for the mother, so encourage the mother to do the best she can without making her feel guilty if a push slips out.
9. Light or 1+ meconium can be managed by thorough **suctioning of the mouth and then the nose at delivery of the head** before the first breath. (Suctioning the nose may stimulate a breath with resulting aspiration of mouth contents.)
10. 2+ or 3+ meconium requires *thorough* suctioning of the mouth and then the nose at delivery of the head.

11. After the body delivers, without stimulating the infant, the individual experienced in neonatal intubation should take the infant and immediately visualize and suction the trachea. This must be accomplished in 1 minute or less. The baby can then be gently dried and stimulated to breathe and resuscitated if necessary as described on page 62.

Signs of Possible Fetal Hypoxia

Description

Fetal hypoxia is presumed present when the various means of ascertaining fetal well-being (FHTs, fetal movement, clear amniotic fluid) are not reassuring.

Clinical Signs and Diagnostic Findings

FHT abnormalities as described on page 9.
Lack of fetal movement.
If the bag of waters is ruptured and meconium is present (green or yellow tinting of the fluid), it must be assumed that the fetus has been and may continue to be compromised.

Nursing Actions

1. If labor and delivery is in-house, transfer immediately.
2. If the membranes are ruptured, an immediate vaginal examination should be conducted to rule out a prolapsed cord.
3. Turn the mother on her left side. If the fetal heart is bradycardic (<100), try alternative positions (right side, back) if left side-lying does not improve the rate. Try the knee-chest position, which takes pressure off the presenting part.
4. Administer supplemental oxygen.
5. Establish large-bore intravenous line with crystalloid fluid and run rapidly.
6. Explain procedures, findings, and plan to mother and her significant others calmly and honestly.

7. If the sign of concern is meconium, see page 72.
8. If a severe bradycardia cannot be corrected, the fetus is of a viable age, and vaginal delivery is not imminent, an immediate cesarean section is indicated. The decision regarding transfer must weigh the speed and safety of a cesarean section at your facility and the viability of a neonatal transfer team coming to accept the infant at delivery against the speed with which the patient could be transferred to a receiving hospital. Should the patient be transferred, call the receiving hospital so that staff there can have the operating room and team prepared.

Prolapsed Umbilical Cord

Description

A prolapsed umbilical cord occurs when the membranes are ruptured and the umbilical cord presents at the cervix or has dropped through the cervix ahead of the presenting part, being compressed between the cervix and the presenting part. **Compression of the umbilical cord deprives the fetus of oxygen. Only immediate delivery can prevent fetal brain damage or death.** Umbilical cord prolapse occurs once in every 275 deliveries (Dildy and Clark, 1993).

Clinical and Diagnostic Findings

The cord may be seen coming from the vagina, or it may be felt on vaginal examination as a pulsing hose-like object or as a limp, soft object.
The mother may report cessation of movement.
The FHTs may be nonreassuring (see p. 9).
If the membranes are ruptured, meconium may be present in the amniotic fluid (see p. 72).

Nursing Actions

1. If the cord is identified outside the vagina, a person should immediately glove, place a hand in the vagina, and gently push the presenting part up off the cord and cervix. If

the cord was identified during a vaginal examination, the examiner should immediately lift the presenting part off the cord and the cervix. **The examiner should not remove his/her hand from the presenting part until the infant is delivered.**

2. Assist the mother into the **knee-chest** position, which also minimizes the weight of the fetus on the cord.

3. Some practitioners wrap the cord in warm saline-soaked sterile sponges, others replace the cord into the vagina, and others may attempt to replace the cord into the uterus. Be prepared to assist in these strategies (Dildy and Clark, 1993).

4. Administer supplemental high-flow **oxygen.**

5. If labor and delivery is in-house, transfer immediately.

6. Initiate large-bore intravenous line with crystalloid fluids and **give fluids rapidly.**

7. In the case of a limp umbilical cord, ultrasonic determination of fetal demise must be made before measures are discontinued (Dildy and Clark, 1993).

8. **Immediate cesarean section** is indicated. The speed and safety of a cesarean in your facility and the viability of using a neonatal transport team must be weighed against transfer to a receiving hospital.

9. Insert an indwelling urinary catheter. The management plan may include the instillation of 500 to 700 mL normal saline into the bladder to elevate the presenting part while awaiting surgery (Cunningham et al., 1993).

10. **Exception:** If delivery can be accomplished in the next 1 to 3 minutes, have the mother push and deliver the infant over the cord. Be prepared for a baby that needs resuscitation.

Shoulder Dystocia

Description

Shoulder dystocia occurs when the head of the infant is born, the cord is drawn into the pelvis and is compressed, but the shoulders become wedged into the pelvis and cannot be delivered. Shoulder dystocia may be associated with significant fetal morbidity and mortality. The incidence of shoulder dystocia in one study was 0.15% among fetuses weighing greater than 2500 g and 1.7% among those fetuses weighing greater than 4000 g (Cunningham et al., 1993). Shoulder dystocia is caused by fetal macrosomia. Maternal obesity, diabetes, and postterm pregnancy predispose to fetal macrosomia. Shoulder dystocia often occurs after a prolonged second stage or after obstetrical interventions to facilitate delivery of the head (e.g., forceps) and is rarely seen in the E.D. Maternal consequences include an increased incidence of postpartum hemorrhage (from uterine atony as well as from vaginal and cervical lacerations) and puerperal infection.

Once it is evident that delivery of the shoulders cannot be effected following delivery of the head, the deliverer:

1. Checks the position of the fetal shoulders. Inserting two fingers of one hand in front of one fetal shoulder and two fingers of the other hand behind the other fetal shoulder, the fetal shoulders are rotated into the slightly **oblique anteroposterior diameter,** and delivery is attempted again (Fig. 3–6).
2. **Call for obstetrical and pediatric help. Be prepared to resuscitate the infant.**
3. **Bladder is emptied** with a urinary catheter.
4. A large median **episiotomy** is cut.
5. Assist mother to **McRobert's** position (knees drawn to chest) (Fig. 3–7A).
6. An assistant, standing on a stool, should apply **pressure directly above the pubic bone** in a downward direction, holding through subsequent delivery attempts (Fig. 3–7B).
7. Delivery is attempted again, by downward traction on the head.
8. If unable to deliver, fingers are placed behind and in front of fetal shoulders as described in no. 1, the shoulders are rotated 180 degrees (**Woods maneuver**), and delivery is attempted again (Fig. 3–7C).
9. The **posterior fetal hand** is grasped by reaching in along the neck. The hand is swept across the fetal chest and pulled out, delivering the

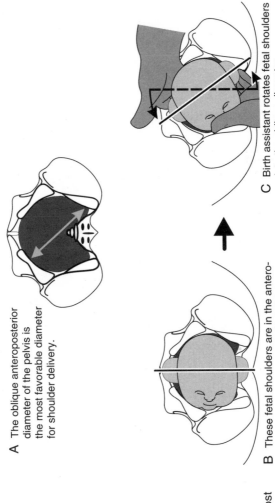

A The oblique anteroposterior diameter of the pelvis is the most favorable diameter for shoulder delivery.

B These fetal shoulders are in the antero-posterior diameter and will deliver more easily if rotated to the oblique.

C Birth assistant rotates fetal shoulders into the oblique diameter.

Figure 3–6. The most favorable pelvic diameter for shoulder delivery.

posterior shoulder; then the delivery is
completed.

10. If unable to deliver, deliberately **fracture the
anterior clavicle** by pressing it against the
maternal pubic bone. (The fracture heals
rapidly and is less serious than other sequelae.)

11. The **Zavanelli maneuver,** finally, is attempted.
The baby's head is placed in occiput anterior or
occiput posterior position, and slowly replaced
into the uterus. Administer 0.25 mg terbutaline
subcutaneously, and perform an emergency
cesarean section. The speed and safety of a
cesarean at your facility, possibly using a
neonatal transport team, must be weighed
against the speed with which the patient can be
transferred to a receiving hospital with an
obstetrical department. Call the receiving
hospital so that they can be ready to operate
immediately.

12. After delivery (by any method), **observe the
mother carefully for postpartum hemorrhage.**
Anticipate administration of prophylactic
antibiotics.

McRobert's position

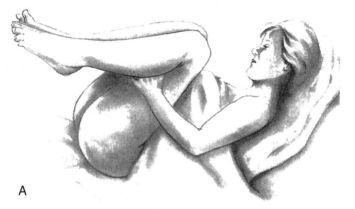

A

Figure 3–7. Strategies for management of shoulder dystocia.
A, McRobert's position.

Illustration continued on following page

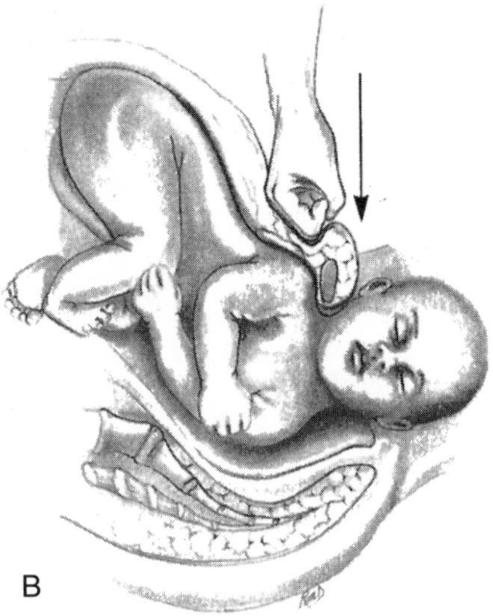

Suprapubic pressure

B

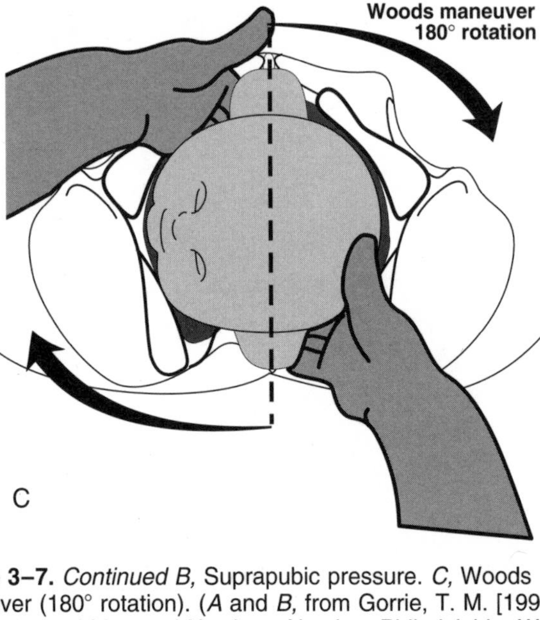

**Woods maneuver
180° rotation**

C

Figure 3–7. *Continued B,* Suprapubic pressure. *C,* Woods maneuver (180° rotation). (*A* and *B,* from Gorrie, T. M. [1994]. Foundations of Maternal Newborn Nursing. Philadelphia: W. B. Saunders, p. 741).

COMPLICATIONS OF THE PUERPERIUM

Mastitis

Description

Mastitis is inflammation of the mammary gland. It usually occurs after the first week and more commonly after the third to fourth week postpartum. The most common causative organism is *Staphylococcus aureus.* The incidence is 5% among lactating mothers (Sammons, 1990).

Differential Diagnoses

Differential diagnoses include breast engorgement (occurs in the first few days postpartum, rarely causes a fever >38.5°C or 101°F, and lasts no longer than 24 to 48 hours [Cunningham et al., 1993]); other causes of fever such as endometritis, thrombophlebitis, viral syndrome, pyelonephritis, or cystitis; a clogged but uninfected milk duct; breast abscess; or other breast disease, such as inflammatory carcinoma.

Clinical and Diagnostic Findings

Hard, swollen, warm, red, tender, and painful breast.
Crack or abrasion of nipple common.
Fever, chills.
Elevated pulse.
Malaise.

Nursing Actions

1. Take vital signs.
2. Anticipate and assist with examination of breasts and other procedures deemed necessary to rule out other causes of fever.
3. Draw blood for CBC and collect other specimens required to rule out other diagnoses.
4. Ultrasound may be required to rule out breast abscess (which would require surgical incision and drainage).
5. Administer acetaminophen (Tylenol) for fever and analgesia for pain as ordered.

6. Depending on the severity of infection, anticipate the prescription of oral antibiotics and discharge to home or admission to the hospital for intravenous antibiotic therapy. The mother should be encouraged to continue nursing frequently on both breasts (Sammons, 1990). Should hospital admission be necessary, arrangements should be made for the infant to room in.

Disposition

When discharged home, the patient should be instructed to increase oral fluids, rest, take acetaminophen for discomfort, consult a lactation consultant for preventive breast-feeding techniques (e.g., positioning), and call her health care provider if no relief is experienced in 24 to 36 hours.

Postpartum Hemorrhage

Description

Postpartum hemorrhage is defined as more than 500 mL blood loss after delivery. The bleeding may come from an episiotomy, a vaginal or cervical laceration, or an uncontracted uterus. Possible causes of uterine atony include a full bladder; undelivered placental fragments or pieces of membranes; or uterine "exhaustion" as a result of, for example, a precipitous labor, a prolonged labor, or a macrosomic infant. The woman who has had five or more children and the woman who has a history of postpartum hemorrhage are at particular risk for postpartum hemorrhage.

Nursing Actions

1. In mild cases, a woman who plans to breast-feed should attempt to nurse the baby. This releases natural oxytocin and slows the bleeding.
2. The bladder should be emptied with a urinary catheter if necessary.
3. Assist in massage of the uterus (which causes it to contract).

4. Anticipate order for Pitocin 10 units IM and Pitocin 10 to 40 units in 1000 mL lactated Ringer's solution running wide open.
5. Assist in visualization of the cervix and vagina to identify any bleeding lacerations. If they are identified, repair is usually done with 2–0 or 3–0 chromic or Vicryl suture.
6. Anticipate bimanual compression by the deliverer if bleeding cannot be controlled (Fig. 3–8).
7. If the mother has no history of hypertension, anticipate an order for ergotamine, methylergonovine (Methergine), or carboprost tromethamine (15-methylprostaglandin $F_{2\alpha}$) (Hemabate). Breast-feeding is a relative contraindication for ergotamine because it may inhibit lactation and is excreted in breast milk. If carboprost is used, remember that gastrointestinal symptoms and fever may occur as side effects (see p. 87).

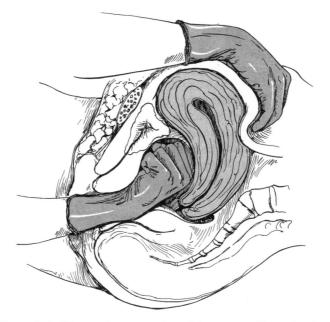

Figure 3–8. Bimanual compression of the uterus. (From Gorrie, T. M. [1994]. Foundations of Maternal Newborn Nursing. Philadelphia: W. B. Saunders, p. 778.)

8. Should shock occur, elevate the legs, administer supplemental oxygen, and order blood to be cross-matched.
9. If bleeding cannot be controlled, the patient must go to surgery for evacuation of the uterus and examination under anesthesia and, possibly, hysterectomy.
10. Once the bleeding is stopped, recheck vaginal bleeding and uterine tone every 5 minutes or more. Document along with vital signs. Once bleeding has been stabilized for an hour, check vital signs, uterine tone, and vaginal bleeding every 15 minutes for at least 1 hour more.
11. Continue to administer Pitocin in the intravenous line after bleeding is controlled, as long as the patient is in the E.D.
12. The patient will be uncomfortable, but narcotics relax the uterus and cannot be given. Other analgesics can be given once the patient is stabilized.
13. As always, explain all procedures, findings, and the plan of management to the patient and her significant others.

Delayed Postpartum Hemorrhage

Description

Delayed postpartum hemorrhage is defined as vaginal bleeding between 24 hours and 6 weeks postpartum. It results primarily from placental site subinvolution, retained products of conception (Cunningham et al., 1993), chronic infection, or previously undiagnosed tumors (Veronikis, 1994). The incidence of delayed postpartum hemorrhage in one study was 0.7% (Cunningham et al., 1993).

Normally after a delivery, vaginal bleeding begins bright red and becomes dark red, brown, yellow, and then clear. It diminishes in quantity. Uterine cramping felt after delivery diminishes and does not return. Variations on this pattern may be explained by increased exertion; however, if the activity level has not increased, the patient is experiencing delayed postpartum hemorrhage.

Clinical and Diagnostic Findings

Large amount of vaginal bleeding greater than 24
  hours after delivery.
Vaginal discharge may have foul odor.
Boggy (indentable) uterus tender to palpation.
Uterus subinvoluted (with bladder empty, the uterus
  should not be palpable above the symphysis pubis
  10 to 14 days after vaginal delivery.
May be febrile with malaise.
Hemoglobin and hematocrit may show anemia or
  may not reflect an acute bleeding episode.

A less acute episode may present with regression of progress in involution as described previously: a return of bright
red bleeding, an increase in the quantity of bleeding, a return
of uterine cramping (or some combination).

Nursing Actions

1. Assess vital signs and vaginal bleeding.
2. For an acute bleeding episode, elevate the legs,
   and administer supplemental oxygen.
3. Initiate a large-bore intravenous line with
   lactated Ringer's solution and run at a rate
   appropriate for the patient's hemodynamic
   condition.
4. Draw blood for CBC, electrolytes, serum hCG,
   and cross-matching. Obtain and send sample for
   urinalysis.
5. Anticipate the administration of intravenous
   oxytocin, carboprost, or methylergonovine or
   ergotamine if the woman is not hypertensive.
   Breast-feeding is also a relative contraindication
   for the administration of ergotamine, which may
   suppress lactation and which is excreted in
   breast milk. If carboprost is used, remember that
   side effects of gastrointestinal disturbances and
   fever may occur.
6. If medical intervention is ineffective, the patient
   must go to surgery for a D&C. Blood should be
   cross-matched for this patient, for whom the
   possibility of hysterectomy is real.

Discharge Instructions

Discharge instructions should include teaching about what is normal (as described previously) and instructions to seek immediate medical attention if symptoms again show regression. The patient may be discharged on a course of oral methylergonovine and antibiotics. Instruct the patient that cramping will occur during the time that she is taking methylergonovine. She should see her prenatal care provider at the end of the course of medication.

DRUGS FOR USE IN OBSTETRICAL EMERGENCIES

Table 3–4 summarizes some emergency drugs that may be used in pregnant patients.

Table 3–4. Emergency Drugs: Considerations in Pregnant Patients

Drugs	Considerations
Alpha agonists (epinephrine)	Uteroplacental vasoconstriction; fetal hypoxia; mild oxytocic
Isoproterenol	Tocolytic, metabolic derangements (glucose, K^+), tachycardia
Atropine	Rapidly crosses placenta; no associated teratogenicity, may or may not affect fetal heart rate
Beta-blockers	Fetal bradycardia, uterine irritability
Dopamine	No adverse effects attributable to drug found in fetuses; may increase or decrease uterine and renal blood flow depending on dose and maternal blood volume
Dobutamine	Little data on use during pregnancy; no identified adverse effects
Nitroprusside	No link with congenital defects; transient fetal bradycardia described; avoidance of prolonged use and monitoring of maternal serum pH, plasma cyanide, and methemoglobin levels recommended
Lidocaine	Maternal seizures, fetal acidosis; fetal central nervous system and cardiovascular depression
Verapamil	Maternal hypotension, uterine atony
Bretylium	Relatively safe

From Esposito, T. J. (1994). Trauma during pregnancy. Emergency Medicine Clinics of North America 12(1), 167–199.

Carboprost Tromethamine (Hemabate)
15-methylprostaglandin $F_{2\alpha}$

Action and Indication

Carboprost tromethamine is an oxytocic that causes uterine contractions. Indicated for postpartum hemorrhage.

Side Effects

Carboprost tromethamine stimulates the smooth muscle of the intestinal tract, causing vomiting or diarrhea (or both) in two thirds of the patients who receive it. Causes transient temperature increases. Causes flushing. May cause transient bronchoconstriction. May raise blood pressure by constricting smooth muscle of the vascular bed.

Contraindications

Patients with active cardiac, pulmonary, renal, or
    hepatic disease.
Undelivered live fetus.

▶ USE WITH CAUTION: *Use with caution in patients with asthma, hypotension or hypertension, diabetes, epilepsy, adrenal disease, or history of previous uterine surgery, including cesarean.*

Dosage

0.25 mg or 250 μg deep IM. May repeat every 15 to 90 minutes, not to exceed eight doses.

Diazoxide (Hyperstat)

Action and Indication

Diazoxide is an antihypertensive that acts by relaxing arteriolar smooth muscle. Recommended for women whose hypertension is refractory to hydralazine. Onset of action 2 to 5 minutes when given IV.

Side Effects

In large doses, diazoxide is associated with fetal compromise and intrauterine death. May cause arrest of labor, maternal and neonatal hyperglycemia, and fluid retention (Probst, 1994). Diazoxide also may displace highly protein-bound drugs, e.g., phenytoin, from their binding sites, increasing the toxicity of those drugs (Probst, 1994).

Dosage

30 mg every 5 to 15 minutes as needed (Probst, 1994; Cunningham et al., 1993; Walker, 1991).

Note: It would be preferable for this drug to be administered with the patient on the fetal monitor in an obstetrical unit. The risk-to-benefit ratio must be weighed.

Ergotamine

Action and Indication

Ergotamine is a uterine muscle stimulant. It also causes constriction of peripheral and cranial blood vessels. Indicated for control of uterine bleeding.

Contraindications

Undelivered live fetus.
Hypertension.
Heart, renal, hepatic, or obliterative vascular disease.

Side Effects

May inhibit lactation.
Present in the breast milk of nursing mothers who
  have received it.
Uterine cramping may result in discomfort.

Dosage

0.2 mg IM; may repeat every 2 to 4 hours; or 0.2 mg orally every 6 to 8 hours for no more than 1 week.

Erythromycin Ophthalmic Ointment (Ilotycin)

Action and Indication

Erythromycin ophthalmic ointment is applied to the eyes of all newborns for prophylaxis of ophthalmia neonatorum due to *Neisseria gonorrhoeae* or *Chlamydia trachomatis*. (Infants born to mothers with clinically evident gonorrhea are treated further according to Centers for Disease Control and Prevention guidelines.)

Side Effects

Eye irritation is seen infrequently.

Dosage

A ribbon of ointment approximately 0.5 to 1.0 cm long from a single-use tube should be instilled into the extended lower eyelid. Do not flush.

Hydralazine (Apresoline)

Action and Indications

Hydralazine is an antihypertensive that acts directly on the vascular wall, causing vasodilation. Most often used first-line drug for preeclampsia (Probst, 1994). Most effective with patient lying flat on her left side in bed. When given IM, the onset of action is 10 to 30 minutes. When given IV, onset of action is 10 minutes with maximum effect in 20 minutes. The duration of action is 6 to 8 hours (Probst, 1994).

Side Effects

Side effects include tachycardia, flushing, nasal congestion, tremors, headache, nausea and vomiting, neonatal thrombocytopenia, reduced placental blood flow, and signs of fetal compromise (Probst, 1994).

Dosage

5 to 10 mg given IV over 1 to 2 minutes every 20 to 30 minutes. If a total dosage of 20 mg has been given without the desired therapeutic effect, another antihypertensive drug should be considered (Probst, 1994).

▶ ALTERNATIVE: *300 mL D5W with 400 mg hydralazine via slow infusion pump; 20 mg given in the first 20 minutes, then the rate is slowed to maintain the desired blood pressure or until the maternal pulse rises to 120 bpm. Dose should not exceed 300 mg/24 hours (Walker, 1991).*

Note: It would be preferable for this drug to be administered with the patient on the fetal monitor in an obstetrical unit. The risk-to-benefit ratio must be weighed.

Labetalol (Trandate)

Action and Indications

Labetalol is an antihypertensive that acts by producing peripheral vasodilation. It has both alpha-adrenergic and beta-adrenergic blocking characteristics; indicated for women whose hypertension is refractory to hydralazine. When given acutely, it reduces blood pressure, heart rate, and peripheral resistance. Onset of action when given IV is 5 to 15 minutes.

Side Effects

Side effects include reactive hypotension (usually seen with continuous infusion, which should then be discontinued immediately [Sibai and Chez, 1994]), tremors, scalp tingling, fetal hypoglycemia, bradycardia, flushing, and nausea (Probst, 1994).

Contraindications

Contraindications are asthma and greater than first-degree heart block.

Dosage

Preferred: Administer 10 to 20 mg IV over 1 to 2 minutes, then 40 mg in 10 minutes, then 80 mg in 10 minutes three times until desired blood pressure achieved or until a total of 300 mg has been given. If desired blood pressure has been achieved, maintain with a continuous infusion of 1 to 2 mg/minute. If blood pressure not controlled after the series of boluses, another drug should be used (Sibai and Chez, 1994).

▶ OR: *Administer 200 mg orally, 600 to 1800 mg/day. Intravenously, administer 50 mg loading dose, then 60 mg/hour (Cunningham, et al., 1993; Walker, 1991).*

▶ OR: *Add 300 mg (60 mL) of labetalol to 240 mL Ringer's lactate to make a 1 mg/mL solution. Start at 1 to 2 mg until hypertension is controlled (not to exceed 1 mg/kg), then reduce to 0.5 mg/minute or less to maintain desired blood pressure. Remember that reactive hypotension occurs more often with continuous infusion (Probst, 1994; Sibai and Chez, 1994).*

Note: It would be preferable for this drug to be administered with the patient on the fetal monitor in an obstetrical unit. The risk-to-benefit ratio must be weighed.

Magnesium Sulfate

Action and Indications

Magnesium sulfate ($MgSO_4$) is a central nervous system depressant and electrolyte replenisher. $MgSO_4$ is used to prevent seizures in the preeclamptic patient and may be used to slow labor because of its tocolytic effects (mechanism unknown). $MgSO_4$ is secreted by the kidney, and decreased urinary output can cause toxicity.

Dosage

Add $MgSO_4$ 10 to 20 g to 1000 mL of a crystalloid solution, calculating the number of milliliters of $MgSO_4$ you will be adding and discarding the same number of milliliters from the plain fluid before mixing to increase accuracy. Administer using an infusion pump:

Loading dose: 4 to 6 g over 20 to 30 minutes
(Gianopoulos, 1994; Probst, 1994).
Maintenance dose: 1 to 3 g/hour (Fadigan, 1994;
Probst, 1994).

Special Instructions

1. When initiating $MgSO_4$ administration, **calcium chloride (CaCl), the antidote of $MgSO_4$, should always be drawn up, labeled, and kept at the bedside.** The dose is 10 mL of 10% CaCl.
2. At the beginning of each hour of $MgSO_4$ administration, observe and chart the patient's

vital signs, FHTs, urine output (by indwelling urinary catheter), and deep tendon reflexes. **If the respirations are less than 12, if urine output is less than 100 mL/4 hours, or if deep tendon reflexes are absent, discontinue MgSO₄ immediately, support respirations, and give CaCl, 10%, 10 mL, slow IV.**

3. Serum Mg level is to be drawn 2 to 4 hours after the initiation of therapy. Therapeutic serum level is 4 to 7 mEq/L (2 to 3 mmol/L). Toxicity is seen above 7 mEq/L, with loss of deep tendon reflexes at 8 to 10 mEq/L, respiratory depression above 11 mEq/L, and respiratory arrest at 13 mEq/L.

Methyldopa (Aldomet)

Action and Indication

Methyldopa works as an antihypertensive by reducing peripheral resistance following a reduction in sympathetic drive. Used for the patient with chronic hypertension. Acts within 2 to 3 hours of an oral dose, peaks at 4 to 8 hours, and lasts 10 to 12 hours.

Side Effects

Side effects include a small bradycardic effect but little or no alteration in cardiac output, sedation, dry mouth, nasal congestion, depression, and postural hypotension.

Dosage

250 to 1000 mg PO daily (Walker, 1991).

Note: It would be preferable for this drug to be administered with the patient on the fetal monitor in an obstetrical unit. The risk-to-benefit ratio must be weighed.

Methylergonovine Maleate (Methergine)

Action and Indication

Methylergonovine is an ergot that acts directly on the uterine muscle to increase the frequency and strength of uterine contractions. Indicated for prevention and control of postpartum hemorrhage. Onset of action is immediate after IV administration, 2 to 3 minutes after IM administration, and 5 to 10 minutes after oral administration.

Contraindications

Hypertension
Preeclampsia/eclampsia
Undelivered live fetus

Dosage

Oral: 1 tablet three to four times per day for a
    maximum of 7 days.
IM: 0.2 mg (= 1 mL) after delivery of the anterior
    shoulder, after delivery of the placenta, or during
    the puerperium. May repeat every 2 to 4 hours.
IV: Same dosage as IM.
    When given IV, may cause sudden hypertension and
    cerebrovascular accident. If essential as a life-saving
    measure, give slowly over at least 1 minute with
    careful blood pressure monitoring.

Naloxone (Narcan)

Action and Indications

Naloxone is a narcotic antagonist indicated for respiratory depression of mother or baby that may be drug-related.

Precautions

Until naloxone reverses any narcotic effect, provide ABCs. Will cause withdrawal symptoms in the neonate who has been passively addicted in utero. Withdrawal symptoms include vomiting, diaphoresis, tachycardia, seizures, tremulousness, hypertension, serum glucose abnormalities, and cardiac arrest.

Dosage

Mother: 5 mg IV

Neonate: 0.01 mg/kg (packaged as neonatal Narcan
with concentration 0.02 mg/mL) to a maximum
dose of 0.4 mg.

Dose will need to be repeated if length of action of narcotic
exceeds that of naloxone.

Nifedipine (Procardia)

Action and Indications

Nifedipine is an antihypertensive that acts by inhibiting extra-
cellular calcium influx into cells, causing vascular smooth muscle relaxation and a decrease in peripheral resistance. Has a
tocolytic effect (i.e., slows uterine contractions). Onset of
action when given orally or sublingually is 20 to 30 minutes
with the effect lasting 3 to 4 hours or longer (Probst, 1994).
Onset of action given orally or sublingually is 10 to 20 minutes.

Side Effects

Side effects include inhibition of labor, headache, nausea,
tachycardia, and flushing.

Precautions

**Action is potentiated by MgSO$_4$; may result in precipitous
and severe hypotension.**

Dosage

10 mg four times a day orally or sublingually; may repeat
every 20 to 30 minutes (Probst, 1994; Cunningham et al.,
1993; Walker, 1991).

Note: It would be preferable for this drug to be administered
with the patient on a fetal monitor in an obstetrical unit. The
risk-to-benefit ratio must be weighed.

Oxytocin (Pitocin)

Action and Indications

Oxytocin is synthetic oxytocin, the pituitary hormone that
stimulates uterine contractions. Indicated in the E.D. to assist

in controlling uterine bleeding after delivery of a pregnancy of any gestation. The onset of action when given IV is almost immediate. The half-life is only 1 to 6 minutes. When given IM, the uterus should respond within 3 to 5 minutes, with a half-life of 2 to 3 hours.

Contraindications

Oxytocin **should not be administered with a live fetus in the uterus unless the patient is on the fetal monitor in a labor and delivery unit.**

Side Effects

Side effects include uterine cramping and pain. Analgesia can be considered, keeping in mind that narcotics relax the uterus and nonnarcotic agents may be more appropriate.

Dosage

With intravenous line in place: 1000 mL lactated
    Ringer's with 10 to 40 units oxytocin over 1 hour.
    Repeat as needed until arrival at an obstetrical
    unit. If bleeding stabilizes, slow the intravenous line
    to 125 mL/hour.
No intravenous line in place: While establishing
    intravenous line, administer 10 units oxytocin IM.

$Rh_0(D)$ Immune Globulin (RhoGAM, Rhesonativ, Gamulin Rh, HypRho-D) (HypRho-D Mini Dose, MICRhoGAM, Mini-Gamulin Rh)

Actions and Indications

$Rh_0(D)$ immune globulin is a solution containing human IgG antibodies to the Rh factor used to prevent the sensitization of Rh-negative individuals exposed to Rh-positive RBCs (see p. 46). It **does not** transmit hepatitis B, HIV, or other viral diseases (Doan-Wiggins, 1994). $Rh_0(D)$ immune globulin attaches to any fetal RBCs in the maternal circulation and traps them in the spleen preventing the maternal immune system from forming antibodies to the Rh antigen. Indicated after delivery, after any type of abortion, ectopic pregnancy, amniocentesis, chorionic villus sampling, catastrophic or noncatastrophic trauma.

Contraindications

Contraindications are previous reaction to human globulin and preexisting Rh sensitization.

Dosage

The regular dose is 300 μg, which protects against 15 mL of Rh-positive packed RBCs. The microdose is 50 μg, which protects against 2.5 mL of packed RBCs and is indicated for gestations of 12 weeks or less. When fetomaternal hemorrhage may exceed 15 mL, the Kleihauer-Betke test is done on maternal serum and the dose is calculated accordingly. Is best administered as soon as possible after the event and before 72 hours. Should more time have transpired, however, it is worth giving the globulin anyway.

Terbutaline (Brethine)

Action and Indications

Terbutaline is a beta-adrenergic receptor agonist, bronchodilator, and uterine muscle relaxant. Indicated for premature labor.

Contraindications

Contraindications are active vaginal bleeding, fetal distress, lethal fetal anomaly, acute chorioamnionitis, maternal hemodynamic compromise, preeclampsia, severe intrauterine growth retardation, and fetal death.

Relative contraindications include chronic hypertension, stable placenta previa, mild abruptio placentae, maternal heart disease, and cervical dilation greater than 5 cm.

Side Effects

Maternal heart rate increases. The mother may experience palpitations, cardiac arrhythmias, and electrolyte and serum

glucose abnormalities. Pulmonary edema and myocardial in-
farction have occurred. Fetal heart rate also increases, and
fetal hyperglycemia can occur.

Dosage

Subcutaneous: Initially give 0.25 to 0.50 mg. If no
  response, may repeat in 30 minutes. Maintain with
  0.25 to 0.50 mg every 2 hours until desired effect
  achieved, until maternal side effects are intolerable,
  or to a maximum dose of 30 mg/day.
Intravenous: Begin at 5 to 10 μg/minute increasing
  every 20 minutes by 5 to 10 μg/minute to a
  maximum dose of 25 μg/minute.
Oral: The patient is usually weaned from the
  subcutaneous or IV routes and placed on oral
  terbutaline at 2.5 to 5.0 mg every 4 to 6 hours.

Vitamin K (AquaMEPHYTON)

Action and Indication

Vitamin K is a clotting factor. Administered to newborn
to prevent hemorrhagic disease of the newborn (most impor-
tantly, intracerebral bleeding) in the first week of life when
clotting factors are diminished because of the fetal liver re-
quiring approximately 1 week of extrauterine life to be fully
functioning.

Side Effects

Vitamin K may contribute to neonatal jaundice but is usually
judged to be worthwhile on a risk-to-benefit basis.

Dosage

0.5 to 1.0 mg IM within 1 hour of birth (use anterior thigh
for injection).

REFERENCES

Abbott, J. (1994). Medical illness during pregnancy. Emergency Medicine Clinics of North America. 12(1), 115–128.

American Academy of Pediatrics Committee on Drugs. (1994). The transfer of drugs and other chemicals into human milk. Pediatrics. 93(1), 137–150.

American College of Obstetricians and Gynecologists (ACOG). (1985). Teratology. ACOG Technical Bulletin. Washington: American College of Obstetricians and Gynecologists.

Blair, F. A., and Hall, M. N. (1994). The nursing process: assessment and priority setting. In Klein, A. R., et al. (Eds.), Emergency Nursing Core Curriculum (pp. 3–23). Philadelphia: W. B. Saunders.

Cefalo, R. C. (1996). Postexposure rabies vaccination during pregnancy: Effect on 202 women and their infants. Comment. *Obstetrical and Gynecological Survey,* 51(1), 3.

Chameides, L., and Hazinski, M. F. (Eds.) (1994). Textbook of Pediatric Advanced Life Support. Dallas: American Heart Association and American Academy of Pediatrics.

Chhabra, R. S., Brion, L. P., Castro, M., Freundlich, L., and Glaser, J. H. (1993). Comparison of maternal sera, cord blood, and neonatal sera for detecting presumptive congenital syphilis: Relationship with maternal treatment. Pediatrics. 91(1), 88–101.

Cunningham, F. G., MacDonald, P. C., and Gant, N. F. (1989). Williams Obstetrics (18th ed.). Norwalk, CT: Appleton & Lange.

Cunningham, F. G., et al. (1993). Williams Obstetrics (19th ed.). Norwalk, CT: Appleton & Lange.

Dildy, G. A., and Clark, S. L. (1993). Umbilical cord prolapse. Contemporary OB/GYN. 38(11), 23–32.

Doan-Wiggins, L. (1994). Drug Therapy for Obstetric Emergencies. Emergency Medicine Clinics of North America. 12(1), 257–272.

Esposito, T. J. (1994). Trauma during pregnancy. Emergency Medicine Clinics of North America. 12(1), 167–199.

Fadigan, A. B., Sealy, D. P., and Schneider, E. F. (1994). Preeclampsia: Progress and puzzle. American Family Physician. 49(4), 849–856.

Gabbe, S. G., Niebyl, J. R., and Simpson, J. L. (1991). Obstetrics: Normal and Problem Pregnancies (2nd ed.) New York: Churchill Livingstone.

Ghidini, A., and Romero, R. (1994). Premature rupture of membranes: When it occurs in second trimester. Contemporary OB/GYN. 39(8), 66–80.

Gianopoulos, J. G. (1994). Emergency complications of labor and delivery. Emergency Medicine Clinics of North America. 12(1), 201–217.

Jehle, D., Krause, R., and Brain, G. R. (1994). Ectopic pregnancy. Emergency Medicine Clinics of North America. 12(1), 55–69.

Khan, N. S., and Luten, R. C. (1994). Neonatal resuscitation. Emergency Medicine Clinics of North America. 12(1), 239–255.

Martens, K. A. (1994). Sexually transmitted and genital tract infections during pregnancy. Emergency Medicine Clinics of North America. 12(1), 91–112.

Probst, B. D. (1994). Hypertensive disorders of pregnancy. Emergency Medicine Clinics of North America. 12(1), 73–89.

Redman, C. W. G., and Roberts, J. M. (1993). Management of pre-eclampsia. The Lancet. 341:1451–1454.

Sammons, L. N. (1990). Mastitis. In Star, W. L., et al. (Eds.), Ambulatory Obstetrics: Protocols for Nurse Practitioners/ Nurse-Midwives (2nd ed.). San Francisco: School of Nursing, University of California, San Francisco.

Sammons, L. N. (1990). Substance abuse. In Star, W. L., et al. (Eds.), Ambulatory Obstetrics: Protocols for Nurse Practitioners/Nurse-Midwives. San Francisco: School of Nursing, University of California, San Francisco.

Sheehy, S. B., McCall, P., and Varvel, P. (1992). Obstetric and gynecologic emergencies. In Sheehy, S. B. (Ed.), Emergency Nursing. Principles and Practice (3rd ed.) (pp. 631–648). St. Louis: Mosby-Year Book, Inc.

Sibai, B. M. (1991). Management of preeclampsia. Clinics in Perinatology. 18(4), 793–808.

Sibai, B. M., and Chez, R. A. (1994). Labetalol for intrapartum hypertension. Clinical dialogue. Contemporary OB/GYN. 39(8), 37–38.

Sibai, B. M., and Mabie, W. C. (1991). Hemodynamics of preeclampsia. Clinics in Perinatology. 18(4), 727–747.

Star, W. L. (1990). Group B streptococcus. In Star, W. L., Shannon, M. T., Sammons, L. N., Lommel, L. L., and Gutierrez, Y. (Eds.), Ambulatory Obstetrics: Protocols for Nurse Practitioners/Nurse-Midwives (2nd ed.) San Francisco: School of Nursing, University of California, San Francisco.

Stone, J. L., et al. (1994). Risk factors for severe preeclampsia. Obstetrics and Gynecology. 83(3), 357–361.

Varney, H. (1987). Nurse-Midwifery (2nd ed.). Boston: Blackwell Scientific Publications.

Veronikis, D. K., and O'Grady, J. P. (1994). What to do—or not do—for postpartum hemorrhage. Contemporary OB/GYN. 39(8), 11–34.

Walker, J. J. (1991). Hypertensive drugs in pregnancy. Antihypertension therapy in pregnancy, preeclampsia, and eclampsia. Clinics in Perinatology. 18(4), 845–867.

Zuspan, F. P. (1991). New concepts in the understanding of hypertensive diseases during pregnancy. An overview. Clinics in Perinatology. 18(4), 653–659.

APPENDICES

APPENDIX A

Breast Engorgement

Description. Engorgement occurs as a result of the hormone prolactin, which is released after delivery to initiate lactation. Milk accumulation and stasis, increased vascularity and congestion, and lymphatic stasis may occur on approximately the third day postpartum and last 24 to 48 hours. **Medications once prescribed to bottle-feeding mothers to prevent breast engorgement have been associated with serious side effects and should no longer be used.**

Clinical and Laboratory Findings

Patient is 2 to 3 days postpartum and may or may not be lactating.

Breasts enlarge and become firm, hard, warm, painful, and tender. Veins are easily visible through the skin. The skin may be tight, shiny, and reddened. The symptoms are generalized over both breasts.

Fever may occur; rarely greater than 38.5°C or 101°F.

Symptoms rarely last more than 24 to 48 hours.

Nursing Actions

1. **Lactating mother:** Instruct the mother to wear a firmly supportive bra. Before nursing, a warm shower or warm compresses to the breasts with massage facilitate milk flow. If the baby is having trouble latching on because of the hardness of the breast, a small amount of milk can be hand-expressed to soften the area behind the nipple. The mother should nurse the baby on demand, at least every 2 hours, for at least 15 minutes on each side, starting with a different side at each nursing. She should be drinking lots of fluids and should be resting when not taking care of the baby. She can use acetaminophen (Tylenol) for discomfort.

2. **Bottle-feeding mother:** Instruct the mother to wear a firmly supportive bra. Alternatively a binder can be used or a towel wrapped tightly and pinned together. The mother should apply

ice to the breast and should not apply heat to the breasts. She should *not* express any milk in an attempt to lessen the engorgement, as the breast works on a supply-and-demand basis, and this encourages milk production. In the shower, she should keep her back to the water to avoid stimulation of the nipples and heat to the breasts. She can minimize oral fluids for the engorgement period. She can use acetaminophen or ibuprofen for pain relief. She should be told that the worst discomfort lasts approximately 24 hours.

APPENDIX B

Culdocentesis

Description and Indication. Culdocentesis is aspiration of fluid from the rectovaginal cul-de-sac. When the patient is stable and ultrasound is not available, this procedure may be used to rule out ectopic pregnancy (Jehle et al., 1994).

Procedure. The patient is positioned on a pelvic examination table with legs in stirrups and the head of the bed elevated to a sitting position so that fluid in the peritoneum collects in the rectovaginal cul-de-sac. A speculum is placed in the vagina, and the cervix is grasped with a tenaculum (patient feels a cramp). The vagina is cleansed with povidone-iodine (Betadine) and a needle is inserted through the posterior fornix of the vaginal wall into the rectovaginal cul-de-sac, which is then aspirated (Fig. B–1).

Interpretation of Findings

A dry aspiration has no diagnostic value. The withdrawal of nonsanguineous fluid is a negative result. Aspiration of blood is considered positive. **Note: A negative test does not rule out an unruptured ectopic pregnancy.**

Nursing Actions

1. Explain procedure to the patient.
2. Place patient in upright lithotomy position.
3. Assist with the procedure.
4. Offer support to the patient, anticipating discomfort when the tenaculum is applied to the cervix and when the needle is placed through the vaginal wall.

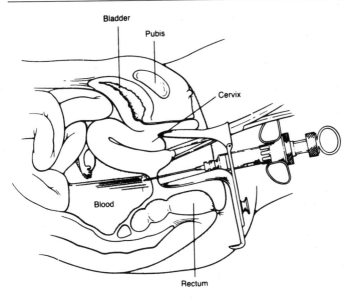

Figure B–1. Culdocentesis. (From Vander Salm [1979]. *Atlas of bedside procedures.* Boston: Little Brown & Co., p. 310.)

APPENDIX C

Conversion Tables

Centimeters to Inches

Centi-meters	30	40	50	60
0 1	11¾ inches 12¼	15¾ inches 16¼	19¾ inches 20	23½ inches 24
2 3	12½ 13	16½ 17	20½ 21	24½ 24¾
4 5	13½ 13¾	17¼ 17¾	21¼ 21¾	25¼ 25½
6 7	14¼ 14½	18 18½	22 22½	26 26½
8 9	15 15¼	19 19¼	22¾ 23¼	26¾ 27¼

Grams to Pounds

| grams ▲ | | less than 1000 | | 1000 | | 2000 | | 3000 | | 4000 | |
| kilograms ▲ | | less than 1 | | 1 | | 2 | | 3 | | 4 | |
grams ▼	kilograms ▼	lb	oz	lb	oz	lb	oz	lb	oz	lb	oz
0	0	0	0	2	3	4	7	6	10	8	13
50	.05	0	2	2	5	4	8	6	12	8	15
100	.1	0	4	2	7	4	10	6	13	9	1
150	.15	0	5	2	9	4	12	6	15	9	2
200	.2	0	7	2	10	4	14	7	1	9	4
250	.25	0	9	2	12	4	15	7	3	9	6

Table continued on following page

Grams to Pounds

grams	kilograms	less than 1000 (less than 1)		1000 (1)		2000 (2)		3000 (3)		4000 (4)	
grams ▼	kilograms ▼	lb	oz	lb	oz	lb	oz	lb	oz	lb	oz
300	.3	0	11	2	14	5	1	7	4	9	8
350	.35	0	12	3	0	5	3	7	6	9	9
400	.4	0	14	3	1	5	5	7	8	9	11
450	.45	1	0	3	3	5	6	7	10	9	13
500	.5	1	2	3	5	5	8	7	11	9	15

550	.55	1	3	3	7	5	10	7	13	10	0
600	.6	1	5	3	8	5	12	7	15	10	2
650	.65	1	7	3	10	5	13	8	1	10	4
700	.7	1	9	3	12	5	15	8	3	10	6
750	.75	1	10	3	14	6	1	8	4	10	8
800	.8	1	12	4	0	6	3	8	6	10	9
850	.85	1	14	4	1	6	5	8	8	10	11
900	.9	2	0	4	3	6	6	8	9	10	13
950	.95	2	1	4	5	6	8	8	11	10	15

Appendix D

Determination of Rupture of Membranes

Description and Indication. The amniotic membranes may rupture grossly with a large amount of fluid in evidence, or they may develop a small leak and the woman may complain that her underwear is repeatedly getting wet. In either case, incontinence of urine or other vaginal secretions must be ruled out. In the case of a slow leak, these tests are reassurance but not absolute proof that the membranes are intact.

Procedure. A sterile speculum examination is done, using minimal or preferably no lubricant. The following signs are observed:

1. Is there fluid pooled in the vaginal vault, and can fluid be seen coming from the cervical os?
2. Litmus or Nitrazine paper turns bright blue in the presence of amniotic fluid. (Blood and cervical mucus also cause a bright blue result.)
3. A swab dipped in fluid is used to make a slide. The slide is allowed to dry thoroughly. Under microscopic examination, a characteristic fern pattern is noted when amniotic fluid, with its salt content, is present. Cervical mucus, however, also dries with a ferning effect (Fig. D–1).

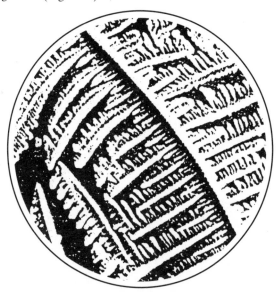

Figure D–1. The ferning pattern seen microscopically when viewing a slide of dried amniotic fluid.

APPENDIX E

Drug Therapy During Pregnancy

Many drugs cross the placental barrier and affect the fetus during pregnancy. During the first trimester, as the fetal organs are developing, the fetus is the most vulnerable for major birth defects. After the first trimester, the effect of environmental factors may be limited to a minimal reduction in organ size or functional defects (ACOG, 1985). Some agents cause major defects if fetal exposure occurs during a specific critical time but cause no harmful effect at another time. There is also a genetically determined threshold of susceptibility to a constant dose of a given drug. Major birth defects are apparent in about 3% of the general population at birth, and the cause of half of these defects is never known.

Many drugs have not been proven safe in pregnancy. Table E–1 lists those drugs that have been proven to be teratogenic.

Table E–1. Documented Teratogens

Agent	Effects	Comments
Antithyroid drugs, e.g., propylthiouracil, iodide, and methimazole (Tapazole)	Hypothyroidism, fetal goiter	Goiter in fetus may lead to malpresentation with hyperextended head. Effect is in part related to dose and duration of therapy
Chemotherapeutic drugs, e.g., methotrexate (Mexate) and aminopterin	Increased risk for spontaneous abortions, various anomalies	These drugs are generally contraindicated for the treatment of psoriasis in pregnancy and must be used with extreme caution in the treatment of malignancy. Most authors indicate that cytotoxic drugs are potentially teratogenic. Effects of aminopterin are well documented. Folic acid antagonists used during the first trimester produce up to a 30% malformation rate in fetuses that survive
Diethylstilbestrol (DES)	Vaginal adenosis, abnormalities of cervix and uterus in females, possible infertility in males and females	Vaginal adenosis is detected in more than 50% of women whose mothers took these drugs before the 9th week of pregnancy. Risk for vaginal adenocarcinoma is low. Males exposed in utero may have a 25% incidence of epididymal cysts, hypotrophic testes, abnormal spermatozoa, and induration of the testes
Lead	Increased abortion rate and stillbirths	Central nervous system development of the fetus may be adversely affected
Lithium	Congenital heart disease, in particular, Ebstein's anomaly	Heart malformations due to first-trimester exposure occur in approximately 2%. Exposure in the last month of gestation may produce toxic effects on the thyroid, kidneys, and neuromuscular systems

Drug	Effects	Notes
(methyl mercury)	spasticity, seizures, blindness	...imester. Exposed individuals include consumers of contaminated grain and fish. Contamination is usually with methyl mercury
Phenytoin (Dilantin)	Growth deficiency, mental retardation, microcephaly, dysmorphic features, hypoplastic nails and distal phalanges	Full syndrome is seen in less than 10% of children exposed in utero; up to 30% have some manifestations. Mild to moderate mental retardation is found in two thirds of children who have severe physical stigmata
Isotretinoin (Accutane)	Increased abortion rate, microtia, nervous system defects, cardiovascular effects, craniofacial dysmorphism, microphthalmos, cleft palate	First trimester exposure may result in approximately 25% anomaly rate
Streptomycin	Hearing loss, VIIIth nerve damage	Animal studies show histologic changes in the inner ear
Tetracycline	Hypoplasia of tooth enamel, incorporation of tetracycline into bone	Drug has no known effect unless exposure occurs in second or third trimester
Thalidomide	Bilateral limb deficiencies—days 27–40, anotia and microtia—days 21–27, other anomalies	Of children whose mothers used thalidomide, 20% show the effect
Trimethadione (Tridione) and paramethadione (Paradione)	Cleft lip or cleft palate, cardiac defects, growth retardation, microcephaly, mental retardation, ophthalmologic abnormalities	Risk for defects or spontaneous abortion is 60–80% with first-trimester exposure. A syndrome including V-shaped eyebrows, low-set ears, high arched palate, and irregular dentition has been identified
Valproic acid (Depakene)	Neural tube defects	Exposure must be before normal closure of neural tube during first trimester to get open defect. Neural tube defects can be diagnosed by alpha-fetoprotein or ultrasound. Incidence of neural tube defects in exposed fetuses is 1–2%

Table continued on following page

Table E–1. Documented Teratogens *Continued*

Agent	Effects	Comments
Drugs and Chemicals		
Alcohol	Growth retardation, mental retardation, microcephaly, reduced size of palpebral fissures, various major and minor malformations	Nutritional deficiency states, smoking, and drug use confound data. Risk due to ingestion of one to two drinks per day (1–2 oz) is not well defined but may cause a small reduction in average birth weight. Fetuses of women who drink six drinks per day (6 oz) are at a 40% risk to show some features of the fetal alcohol syndrome
Androgens	Pseudohermaphroditism in female offspring, advanced genital development in males	Effects are dose dependent and related to stage of embryonic development. Depending on time of exposure, clitoral enlargement or labioscrotal fusion can be produced. The risk related to incidental brief androgenic exposure is minimal
Anticoagulants, e.g., warfarin (Coumadin; Panwarfin) and dicumarol	Hypoplastic nose, bony abnormalities, stippling of secondary epiphyses, broad short hands with shortened phalanges, ophthalmologic abnormalities, intrauterine growth retardation, anomalies of neck, central nervous system defects	Risk for a seriously affected child is considered to be 25% when anticoagulants that inhibit vitamin K are used in the first trimester. Later drug exposure may be associated with spontaneous abortions, stillbirths, central nervous system abnormalities, abruptio placentae, and fetal or neonatal hemorrhaging

From American College of Obstetricians and Gynecologists (ACOG) (1985). Teratology. ACOG Technical Bulletin Number 84. Washington, D.C.: American College of Obstetricians and Gynecologists.

APPENDIX F

Drug Therapy During Lactation

Many drugs taken by the mother either affect her ability to produce milk or are excreted in breast milk to be absorbed by the baby. The American Academy of Pediatrics suggests the following considerations before giving a drug to a lactating woman: (1) Is the drug therapy really necessary? (2) Is there a safer drug? (3) If there is a possibility that the drug may present a risk to the infant, consider measuring the blood concentrations in the nursing infant. (4) Minimize the infant's ingestion of the drug by having the mother take the drug just after she has breast-fed the infant or just before the infant is due for a lengthy sleep period (AAP, 1994). In addition, if necessary, nursing can be interrupted; the breasts are pumped and the milk discarded, the baby is given previously pumped and saved breast milk or formula for the duration of therapy, and nursing is then resumed. Although this approach is undesirable, it is preferable to telling the mother she must discontinue nursing if a particular drug therapy is important.

Tables F–1 through F–6 were published by the American Academy of Pediatrics' Committee on Drugs. They contain the most recent information about the safety of various drugs for the lactating woman and her infant.

Table F–1. Drugs That Are Contraindicated During Breast-Feeding

Drug	Reason for Concern, Reported Sign or Symptom in Infant, or Effect on Lactation
Bromocriptine	Suppresses lactation; may be hazardous to the mother
Cocaine	Cocaine intoxication
Cyclophosphamide	Possible immune suppression; unknown effect on growth or association with carcinogenesis; neutropenia
Cyclosporine	Possible immune suppression; unknown effect on growth or association with carcinogenesis
Doxorubicin*	Possible immune suppression; unknown effect on growth or association with carcinogenesis
Ergotamine	Vomiting, diarrhea, convulsions (doses used in migraine medications)
Lithium	One third to one half therapeutic blood concentration in infants
Methotrexate	Possible immune suppression; unknown effect on growth or association with carcinogenesis; neutropenia
Phencyclidine (PCP)	Potent hallucinogen
Phenindione	Anticoagulant; increased prothrombin and partial thromboplastin time in one infant; not used in United States

*Drug is concentrated in human milk.
From AAP Committee on Drugs. (1994). The transfer of drugs and other chemicals into human milk. Pediatrics. 93(1), 137–150.

Table F–2. Drugs of Abuse: Contraindicated During Breast-Feeding*

Drug Reference	Reported Effect or Reasons for Concern
Amphetamine†	Irritability, poor sleeping pattern
Cocaine	Cocaine intoxication
Heroin	Tremors, restlessness, vomiting, poor feeding
Marijuana	Only one report in literature; no effect mentioned
Nicotine (smoking)	Shock, vomiting, diarrhea, rapid heart rate, restlessness; decreased milk production
Phencyclidine	Potent hallucinogen

*The Committee on Drugs strongly believes that nursing mothers should not ingest any compounds listed in this table. Not only are they hazardous to the nursing infant, but also they are detrimental to the physical and emotional health of the mother. This list is obviously not complete; no drug of abuse should be ingested by nursing mothers even though adverse reports are not in the literature.

†Drug is concentrated in human milk.

From AAP Committee on Drugs. (1994). The transfer of drugs and other chemicals into human milk. Pediatrics. 93(1), 137–150.

Table F–3. Drugs Whose Effect on Nursing Infants Is Unknown but May Be of Concern*

Drug	Reported or Possible Effect
Antianxiety	
Diazepam	None
Lorazepam	None
Midazolam	—
Perphenazine	None
Prazepam†	None
Quazepam	None
Temazepam	—
Antidepressants	
Amitriptyline	None
Amoxapine	None
Desipramine	None
Dothiepin	None
Doxepin	None
Fluoxetine	—
Fluvoxamine	—
Imipramine	None
Trazodone	None
Antipsychotic	
Chlorpromazine	Galactorrhea in adult; drowsiness and lethargy in infant
Chlorprothixene	None
Haloperidol	None
Mesoridazine	None
Chloramphenicol	Possible idiosyncratic bone marrow suppression
Metoclopramide†	None described; dopaminergic blocking agent
Metronidazole	In vitro mutagen; may discontinue breast-feeding 12–24 hr to allow excretion of dose when single-dose therapy given to mother
Tinidazole	See metronidazole

*Psychotropic drugs, the compounds listed under antianxiety, antidepressant, and antipsychotic categories, are of special concern when given to nursing mothers for long periods. Although there are no case reports of adverse effects in breast-feeding infants, these drugs do appear in human milk and thus could conceivably alter short-term and long-term central nervous system function.

†Drug is concentrated in human milk.

From AAP Committee on Drugs. (1994). The transfer of drugs and other chemicals into human milk. Pediatrics. 93(1), 137–150.

Table F–4. Drugs That Have Been Associated with Significant Effects on Some Nursing Infants and Should Be Given to Nursing Mothers with Caution*

Drug	Reported Effect
5-Aminosalicylic acid	Diarrhea (1 case)
Aspirin (salicylates)	Metabolic acidosis (1 case)
Clemastine	Drowsiness, irritability, refusal to feed, high-pitched cry, neck stiffness (1 case)
Phenobarbital	Sedation; infantile spasms after weaning from milk containing phenobarbital, methemoglobinemia (1 case)
Primidone	Sedation, feeding problems
Sulfasalazine (salicylazosulfapyridine)	Bloody diarrhea (1 case)

*Measure blood concentration in the infant when possible.

From AAP Committee on Drugs. (1994). The transfer of drugs and other chemicals into human milk. Pediatrics. 93(1), 137–150.

Table F–5. Maternal Medications Usually Compatible with Breast-Feeding*

Drug	Reported Sign or Symptom in Infant or Effect on Lactation
Acebutolol	None
Acetaminophen	None
Acetazolamide	None
Acitretin	—
Acyclovir†	None
Alcohol (ethanol)	With large amounts drowsiness, diaphoresis, deep sleep, weakness, decrease in linear growth, abnormal weight gain; maternal ingestion of 1 g/kg daily decreases milk ejection reflex
Allopurinol	—
Amoxicillin	None
Antimony	—
Atenolol	None
Atropine	None
Azapropazone (apazone)	—
Aztreonam	None
B_1 (thiamine)	None
B_6 (pyridoxine)	None
B_{12}	None
Baclofen	None
Barbiturate	See Table F–4
Bendroflumethiazide	Suppresses lactation
Bishydroxycoumarin (dicumarol)	None
Bromide	Rash, weakness, absence of cry with maternal intake of 5.4 g/day
Butorphanol	None
Caffeine	Irritability, poor sleeping pattern, excreted slowly; no effect with usual amount of caffeine beverages

Table F–5. Maternal Medications Usually Compatible with Breast-Feeding* Continued

Drug	Reported Sign or Symptom in Infant or Effect on Lactation
Captopril	None
Carbamazepine	None
Carbimazole	Goiter
Cascara	None
Cefadroxil	None
Cefazolin	None
Cefotaxime	None
Cefoxitin	None
Cefprozil	—
Ceftazidime	None
Ceftriaxone	None
Chloral hydrate	Sleepiness
Chloroform	None
Choroquine	None
Chlorothiazide	None
Chlorthalidone	Excreted slowly
Cimetidine†	None
Cisapride	None
Cisplatin	Not found in milk
Clindamycin	None
Clogestone	None
Clomipramine	—
Codeine	None
Colchicine	—
Contraceptive pill with estrogen/progesterone	Rare breast enlargement; decrease in milk production and protein content (not confirmed in several studies)
Cycloserine	None
D (vitamin)	None; follow up infant's serum calcium level if mother receives pharmacological doses

Table continued on following page

Table F–5. Maternal Medications Usually Compatible with Breast-Feeding* *Continued*

Drug	Reported Sign or Symptom in Infant or Effect on Lactation
Danthron	Increased bowel activity
Dapsone	None; sulfonamide detected in infant's urine
Dexbrompheniramine maleate with *d*-isoephedrine	Crying, poor sleeping patterns, irritability
Digoxin	None
Diltiazem	None
Dipyrone	None
Disopyramide	None
Domperidone	None
Dyphylline†	None
Enalapril	—
Erythromycin†	None
Estradiol	Withdrawal, vaginal bleeding
Ethambutol	None
Ethanol (cf. alcohol)	—
Ethosuximide	None, drug appears in infant serum
Fentanyl	—
Flecainide	—
Flufenamic acid	None
Fluorescein	—
Folic acid	None
Gold salts	None
Halothane	None
Hydralazine	None
Hydrochlorothiazide	—
Hydroxychloroquine†	None
Ibuprofen	None
Indomethacin	Seizure (1 case)
Iodides	May affect thyroid activity; see miscellaneous iodine

Table F–5. Maternal Medications Usually Compatible with Breast-Feeding* *Continued*

Drug	Reported Sign or Symptom in Infant or Effect on Lactation
Iodine (povidone-iodine/ vaginal douche)	Elevated iodine levels in breast milk, odor of iodine on infant's skin
Iodine	Goiter; see miscellaneous, iodine
Iopanoic acid	None
Isoniazid	None; acetyl metabolite also secreted; (?) hepatotoxic
K₁ (vitamin)	None
Kanamycin	None
Ketorolac	—
Labetalol	None
Levonorgestrel	—
Lidocaine	None
Loperamide	—
Magnesium sulfate	None
Medroxyprogesterone	None
Mefenamic acid	None
Methadone	None if mother receiving ≤20 mg/24 hr
Methimazole (active metabolite of carbimazole)	None
Methocarbamol	None
Methyldopa	None
Methyprylon	Drowsiness
Metoprolol†	None
Metrizamide	None
Mexiletine	None
Minoxidil	None
Morphine	None; infant may have significant blood concentration
Moxalactam	None
Nadolol†	None

Table continued on following page

Table F–5. Maternal Medications Usually Compatible with Breast-Feeding* *Continued*

Drug	Reported Sign or Symptom in Infant or Effect on Lactation
Nalidixic acid	Hemolysis in infant with glucose-6-phosphate dehydrogenase (G-6-PD) deficiency
Naproxen	—
Nefopam	None
Nifedipine	—
Nitrofurantoin	Hemolysis in infant with G-6-PD deficiency
Norethynodrel	None
Norsteroids	None
Noscapine	None
Oxprenolol	None
Phenylbutazone	None
Phenytoin	Methemoglobinemia (1 case)
Piroxicam	None
Prednisone	None
Procainamide	None
Progesterone	None
Propoxyphene	None
Propranolol	None
Propylthiouracil	None
Pseudoephedrine†	None
Pyridostigmine	None
Pyrimethamine	None
Quinidine	None
Quinine	None
Riboflavin	None
Rifampin	None
Scopolamine	—
Secobarbital	None
Senna	None
Sotalol	—

Table F–5. Maternal Medications Usually Compatible
with Breast-Feeding* Continued

Drug	Reported Sign or Symptom in Infant or Effect on Lactation
Spironolactone	None
Streptomycin	None
Sulbactam	None
Sulfapyridine	Caution in infant with jaundice or G-6-PD deficiency, and ill, stressed, or premature infant; appears in infant's milk
Sulfisoxazole	Caution in infant with jaundice or G-6-PD deficiency, and ill, stressed, or premature infant; appears in infant's milk
Suprofen	None
Terbutaline	None
Tetracycline	None; negligible absorption by infant
Theophylline	Irritability
Thiopental	None
Thiouracil	None mentioned; drug not used in United States
Ticarcillin	None
Timolol	None
Tolbutamide	Possible jaundice
Tolmetin	None
Trimethoprim/ sulfamethoxazole	None
Triprolidine	None
Valproic acid	None
Verapamil	None
Warfarin	None
Zolpidem	None

* Drugs listed have been reported in the literature as having the effects listed or no effect. The word *none* means that no observable change was seen in the nursing infant while the mother was ingesting the compound. It is emphasized that most of the literature citations concern single case reports or small series of infants.

† Drug is concentrated in human milk.

From AAP Committee on Drugs. (1994). The transfer of drugs and other chemicals into human milk. Pediatrics. 93(1), 137–150.

Table F–6. Food and Environmental Agents: Effect on Breast-Feeding

Agent	Reported Sign or Symptom in Infant or Effect on Lactation
Aflatoxin	None
Aspartame	Caution if mother or infant has phenylketonuria
Bromide (photographic laboratory)	Potential absorption and bromide transfer into milk; see Table F–5
Cadmium	None reported
Chlordane	None reported
Chocolate (theobromine)	Irritability or increased bowel activity if excess amounts (16 oz/day) consumed by mother
DDT, benzenehexachlorides, dieldrin, aldrin, hepatachlorepoxide	None
Fava beans	Hemolysis in patient with glucose-6-phosphate dehydrogenase (G-6-PD) deficiency
Fluorides	None
Hexachlorobenzene	Skin rash, diarrhea, vomiting, dark urine, neurotoxicity, death
Hexachlorophene	None; possible contamination of milk from nipple washing
Lead	Possible neurotoxicity
Methyl mercury, mercury	May affect neurodevelopment
Monosodium glutamate	None
Polychlorinated biphenyls and polybrominated biphenyls	Lack of endurance, hypotonia, sullen expressionless facies
Tetrachlorethylene cleaning fluid (perchloroethylene)	Obstructive jaundice, dark urine
Vegetarian diet	Signs of B_{12} deficiency

From AAP Committee on Drugs. (1994). The transfer of drugs and other chemicals into human milk. Pediatrics. 93(1), 137–150.

APPENDIX G

Equipment Lists

Pelvic tray: speculum; optional—sponge forceps with sponges, emesis basin.

Culdocentesis tray: speculum, glass syringe with Iowa trumpet, emesis basin, small cup with sponges, sponge forceps, and tenaculum.

BOA (born out of asepsis) pack: scissors, 2 Kelly clamps, towels, gauze, placenta basin, bulb syringe, optional—needle driver, additional pair scissors, forceps.

Neonatal resuscitation equipment: see Table G–1.

Table G–1. Neonatal Resuscitation Equipment

Gowns, gloves, goggles (for universal precautions)
Towels
Heat source (radiant warmer or heating lamps)
Warmed blankets
Suction with manometer
Self-inflating bag (450–750 mL)
Face masks (premature, newborn, and infant sizes)
Laryngoscope handles (2) with extra batteries and bulbs
Laryngoscope blades (straight 0 and 1)
Medications and fluids
  Epinephrine 1 : 10,000
  Volume expanders (5% albumin, normal saline, lactated
    Ringer's solution)
  Naloxone hydrochloride (1 mg/mL or 0.4 mg/mL)
  Sodium bicarbonate (0.5 mEq/mL—4.2% solution*)
Bulb syringe
Meconium aspirator (for attachment to mechanical suction)
Endotracheal tubes (2.5, 3.0, 3.5) 2 of each
Endotracheal tube stylets
Suction catheters (5-Fr, 8-Fr, 10-Fr), 2 of each
Umbilical catheters (3.5-Fr, 5-Fr)
Syringes (1, 3, 10, 20 mL)
Three-way stopcocks
Feeding tubes (8-Fr, 10-Fr)
Sterile umbilical vessel catheterization tray

* If an 8.4% solution is the only one available, it should be diluted 1 : 1 with sterile water.
From Chameides, L., and Hazinski, M. F. (Eds.) (1994). Textbook of Pediatric Advanced Life Support. Dallas: American Heart Association and American Academy of Pediatrics.

APPENDIX H

Community Resources

The following resources are useful in the provision of emergency care to the pregnant woman. The user is invited to find such agencies in his or her region and enter names and numbers in the space below:

Hotline for women's services:

Centers for women seeking abortion:

Battered women's hotline and/or shelters:

Prenatal care:

Teratogenic counseling hotline:

Support group for parents after miscarriage, stillbirth, or infant death:

INDEX

Note: Page numbers in *italics* refer to illustrations;
page numbers followed by t refer to tables.